MEN'S HEALTH® BEST
ABS

MEN'S HEALTH® BEST
ABS

EDITED BY **JOE KITA**,
MEN'S HEALTH® MAGAZINE

This edition first published in 2005 by
Rodale International Ltd
7–10 Chandos Street
London
W1G 9AD
www.rodale.co.uk

© 2005 Rodale Inc.

"Men's Health®" is a registered trademark of Rodale Inc.

Interior photographs:
Beth Bischoff p. 28, 29, 35, 36, 37, 40, 41, 47, 50, 51, 52, 53, 54, 57, 60, 61, 62, 63, 64, 65, 66, 67, 68, 69, 71 (top, middle), 74, 75, 76 (top), 77, 78, 79, 80, 81 (bottom left, bottom right), 82 (top left, top right), 84 (bottom left, bottom right), 85, 86, 87, 89, 90, 91, 92, 94; Brand X Pictures p. 30; Colin Cooke p. 19; Corbis p. 16, 34, 46; Digital Vision p. 6, 42; Image Source p. 9, 15, 49; Mitchel Gray p. 55, 58, 59, 70, 71 (bottom), 72, 73, 76 (bottom), 81 (top left, top right), 82 (bottom left, bottom right), 83, 84 (top left, top right), 88, 93; Michael Mazzeo p. 22, 23, 24, 25, 26, 33; Photodisc p. 12, 17, 18, 20, 27; Fabrice Trombert p. 56; Craig Zuckerman p. 11.

Printed and bound China.
3 5 7 9 8 6 4

ISBN 978-1-4050-7750-7

Notice
The information in this book is meant to supplement, not replace, proper exercise training. All forms of exercise pose some inherent risks. The editors and publisher advise readers to take full responsibility for their safety and know their limits. Before practising the exercises in this book, be sure that your equipment is well maintained, and do not take risks beyond your level of experience, aptitude, training and fitness.

The exercise and dietary programmes in this book are not intended as a substitute for any exercise routine or dietary regime that may have been prescribed by your doctor. As with all exercise and dietary programmes, you should get your doctor's approval before beginning.

Visit us on the Web at *www.menshealth.co.uk*

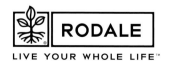

CONTENTS

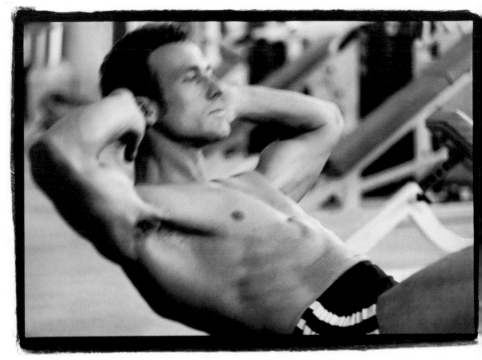

Work your abs just two or three times a week to promote both muscle gain and fat loss.

INTRODUCTION

Abs are everywhere. On the covers of fitness magazines. On late-night television ads and on billboards. The 'six-pack' has become the symbol of the ideal male body type. Do abdominal muscles actually warrant such a place at centre stage in our culture?

Putting aside issues of vanity and/or virility, the muscles of the midsection really are extraordinary, and research is demonstrating that they play a vital role in supporting the body's core and, most remark-able of all, in the body's chemistry. Recent evidence indicates that a strong, lean abdomen is one of the most reliable predictors of wellness.

Study after study shows that the people with the largest waist sizes have the most risk of life-threatening disease. There is strong evidence that a waistline larger than 110 centimetres (40 inches) for men signals significant risk of heart disease and diabetes. Of course, killer abs don't guarantee you a get-out-of-the-hospital-free card, but studies show that by developing a strong abdominal section, you'll reduce body fat and significantly cut the risk factors associated with many diseases, not just heart disease. The incidence of cancer among obese patients is 33 per cent higher than among lean ones, according to a Swedish study. Upper-body obesity is also the most significant risk factor for obstructive sleep apnoea. Are you ready for some more bad news? Fat tissue in your abdomen spurs your body to produce hormones that prompt your cells to divide. More cell division means more opportunities for cell mutations, which means a higher cancer risk.

Now, the good news – strong, lean abs are not only a reliable indicator of good health, they also can improve your sex life. Strong abdominal and lower back muscles give you increased stamina, better erections and can even make your penis appear larger. You may have picked up this book because you thought it would be nice to try for a six-pack. You probably didn't realize it could save your life.

MANAGE YOUR MIDDLE

- Do your abs exercises at the beginning of your workout if you can't pass this test: sit with your feet flat on the floor and your legs bent – as if you had just performed a situp. Then place your fingers behind your ears with your elbows pulled back. Lower yourself to the floor as slowly as possible. If it doesn't take at least five seconds, you need to prioritize your abdominal training.
- Don't be afraid of situps. They increase your range of motion, which makes your abdominals work harder and longer. (Doing crunches on an exercise ball – Swiss ball – or with a rolled-up towel under your lower back has a similar effect.) Just avoid situps with anchored feet, which can hurt your lower back.
- Remember to exhale forcefully at the top of the crunch movement – it forces your abs to work harder.
- Don't work your abdominal muscles every day. Your abs are like any other muscle in your body; train them no more than two or three days a week.
- Don't try to lose your gut just by working your abs (among other things, you need to address diet and nutrition, get aerobic exercise, and strengthen your lower back). It actually takes 250,000 crunches to burn ½ kilogram (1 pound) of fat – that's 100 crunches a day for seven years.

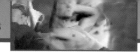

Our mission is simple. We're not promoting fancy dieting gimmicks. We're not looking for amazing weight-loss theories. We haven't invented electronic gizmos or miracle pills. What we have done is create a simple, instinctive and satisfying eating and exercise plan that will flatten any man's midsection.

That means a healthy, muscle-building diet and a variety of exercises. Not just crunches. Too often guys in search of that elusive six-pack have dropped to the ground to tear through endless crunches and situps in the belief that building muscle mass around the waistline would lead to a flat belly. We know now that only a balanced programme – one that includes aerobic exercise, a targeted diet, and weight training that focuses on all major muscle groups including the hips and lower back – will successfully trim your overhang.

The exercises beginning on page 49 recruit many muscles into the abs-building business, bigger muscles in your shoulder, back and legs have to help keep your body balanced. That means a bigger boost in the amount of muscle you build, and also another huge benefit: your abdominal muscles get used to working as nature designed them, at the centre of every complex move you make.

We're loading you up with information about your abdominal muscles because we believe the better you understand the muscles you're working the better you'll recognize and appreciate your progress. We've scoured the sports medicine world for the best stretches and pulled together a selection of more than a dozen crunches and creative exercise variations to keep your workout fresh and effective. We've thrown in pages of recipes and nutrition tips to make sure you stay satisfied with a healthy, balanced diet that's so tasty you won't even notice you're making sacrifices. Basically, we've done our part. Now it's time for you to grab that six-pack.

NO MORE EXCUSES

You think you're too busy to exercise? Try this: for one day, schedule a time to work out, and then stick to it – even if you can exercise for only 10 minutes. At the end of the day, evaluate whether you were any less productive than usual. The answer will probably be no and your favourite excuse will be gone.

PART I:
Abs Essentials

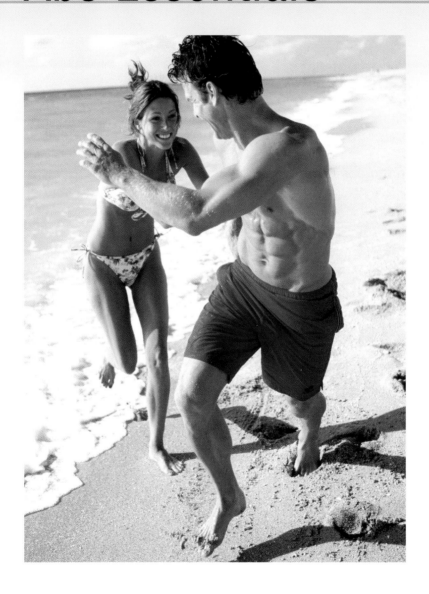

About Your Abs

Your abdominal muscles are a lot like a group of skilled employees. The harder they work, the better they make you look. And vice versa. This is because you use your abs in virtually every movement that matters. Lifting. Running. Jumping. Reproducing. So the stronger they are, the harder and longer you'll be able to play.

The abs-building exercises and workout programmes in this book are designed to work your whole midsection – not just the six-pack muscle (*rectus abdominis*, for you Latin lovers), but also your obliques (at the sides of your waist) and your lower back. Some of the exercises even help strengthen the deep abdominal and lower back muscles that help you sit up straighter when you're working away at the computer. So whether you're bending, twisting or just relaxing, this collection of powerful exercises will ensure that you and your abs will perform better and last longer.

The Transverse Abdominis

Think of the *transverse abdominis* (TA) as a corset. Granted, it's not a very masculine image, but it is apt. Hidden beneath the other three muscles that make up your abs (see Abs Basics, right), the TA wraps around your torso, attaching to your abdominals, pelvis

and ribs. It's a hard-working muscle, too: it supports your whole torso, stabilizes your pelvis, holds your internal organs in place, keeps your gut from flopping over your belt and contributes to proper posture.

Considering how important the TA is, it's surprising how little attention it receives by most people – even those who consider themselves fit. Poor posture is a cause and an effect of ignoring the TA. It's a vicious circle: neglect your TA and your posture suffers. Walk around with poor posture, and you're weakening your TA even further. The result? Muscular imbalances that contribute to back injuries.

What's the answer? Get in touch with your TA. Learn how to engage it during everyday movements (tilt your pelvis forwards and pull your navel in towards your spine) and concentrate on exercises that work the TA. The Bridge (page 74) and Swiss Ball Bridge (page 76) are two good places to start.

ABS BASICS

Meet the four muscle groups that make up your midsection:

Rectus Abdominis:
This is the six-pack muscle that helps your upper body bend (like in a crunch) and also helps keep good posture. It's what people think of when they think of abs.

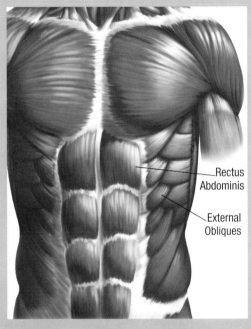

Rectus Abdominis

External Obliques

External Obliques:
These muscles start on the ribs and extend diagonally down the sides of your waist. If a movement happens at your waist, the external obliques are involved. The torso rotation that's key to golf, tennis and hockey is mostly a function of the external obliques. Even the basic crunching motion, attributed to the rectus abdominis (the six-pack muscle), wouldn't be possible without a strong contraction of the external obliques to stabilize the torso.

Internal Obliques (not pictured): These lie between the ribcage and the external obliques, and also extend diagonally down the sides of your waist. Similar to the externals, the internal obliques are involved in torso rotation. You use these muscles when you breathe deeply.

Transverse Abdominis (not pictured): It's a thin muscle that runs horizontally, surrounding your abdomen. It's also known as 'the corset' because it functions as a compressor for the abdomen, keeping everything in place.

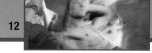

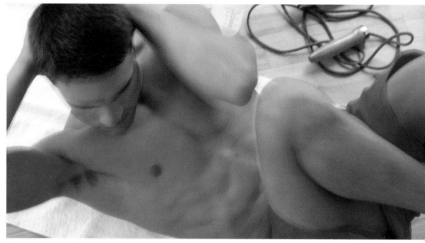

Abs exercises will improve your posture and help protect your back from strains and pulls.

Perfect Your Posture

You can work your abs at any time, even when you're not at the gym. One secret to improving how your belly looks is simply to be aware of it – all day long. Keep your abs taut throughout the day. Even when you're sitting in your car or at your desk, tense your middle as you would at the start of a crunch. Stand or sit up straight and pull your abs in for 60 seconds at a time, at least once an hour. Any time you feel them going slack throughout your day tighten them again. When you're walking, stand tall and picture a cape flowing off your shoulders, superhero-style, to ensure the best posture. Another good trick is to think of your back as a wall and your stomach as a big piece of furniture pushed up against the wall to keep it from buckling.

Remind your abs to look good. You've heard of muscle memory in sports? Well, it works for your abdominal muscles, too. If you consciously keep them firm throughout the day, they'll tend to stay firm even when you're relaxed.

Healthy Abs

The notion that abdominal obesity is the most dangerous kind is not new. Back in the 1940s, the French doctor Jean Vague observed that some obese patients had normal blood chemistry while some moderately overweight patients showed serious abnormalities that predisposed them to heart disease or diabetes. Almost always, the latter patients carried their excess fat around their middles. And, almost always, they were men.

Multiple studies since then have shown that abdominal fat – the cause of the classic apple-shaped body – is more than nature's way of telling you that you'll never become a soap-opera star, newsreader, rock legend or male model. It's a sign of increased risk of weight-related health problems. There are a number of substances your bloated belly secretes to your heart, liver and other vital organs. Among them:

- **Free fatty acids.** Released directly to the liver, they impair your ability to break down insulin, which over time can lead to diabetes.
- **Cortisone.** High levels of this hormone are associated with diabetes and heart disease.
- **PAI-1.** This blood-clotting agent increases your risk of heart attack and stroke.
- **C-Reactive Protein (CRP).** This protein inflames blood vessels, making them more susceptible to artery-clogging plaque.

All these chemicals floating around spells big trouble for big-bellied guys. In a recent study, researchers took 137 men of all ages and sizes and used seven different measurements to determine their risk of cardiovascular disease. The single best sign of multiple heart disease risks? No, it wasn't the mens' family histories or their cholesterol profiles. It was the amount of

ISOLATE YOUR ABS

When you do reverse crunches and hanging knee raises, round your back by rolling your hips and pelvis towards your chest, instead of simply raising your legs. Otherwise, you're mainly working your hip flexors – the muscles at the top of your thighs.

belly fat they carried. By the way, heart disease and diabetes are only two of the ways belly fat can ruin your health. If you count them all up, you'll find at least 39 different diseases associated with abdominal obesity (40, if you include looking terrible with your shirt off).

Support System

Think of your midsection as your body's infrastructure. You don't want a core made of dry, brittle wood or straw. You want one made of solid steel, one that will give you a layer of protection that belly fat never could.

Unlike other muscles in your body, a strong core affects the functioning of the whole body. Whether you ski or wrestle with the kids, your abs are the most essential muscles for protecting you from being injured. The stronger they are, the stronger – and safer – you are.

Since most back pain is related to weak muscles in your trunk, maintaining a strong midsection can help resolve many back issues. The muscles that criss-cross your midsection don't function in isolation; they weave through your torso like a spider's web, even attaching to your spine. When your abdominal muscles are weak, the muscles in your buttocks (your glutes) and along the backs of your legs (your hamstrings) have to compensate for the work your abs should be doing. The effect, besides promoting bad company morale for the muscles picking up the slack, is that it destabilizes the spine and eventually leads to back pain and strain – or even more serious back problems.

When you're playing sports, your abs help stabilize your body during start-and-stop movements, like changing direction on the football pitch or tennis court. If you have weak abs, your joints absorb all the force from those movements. It's like trampoline physics. Jump in the centre, and the mat will absorb your weight and bounce you back in the air. Jump towards the side of the trampoline, where the mat meets the frame, and

SQUAT FOR A SIX-PACK

Squats and deadlifts force your abdominal muscles to do a significant amount of work to maintain your posture.

you'll break the springs. Your body is like a trampoline, with your abs as the centre of the mat and your joints as the supports that hold the mat to the frame. If your abs are strong enough to absorb some shock, you'll function well. If they're not, the force puts far more pressure on your joints than they were built to withstand.

If you play golf or football, or any sport that requires movement (and we're pretty sure that includes all of them), your essential muscle group isn't your chest, biceps or legs. It's your core – the muscles in your torso and hips. Developing core strength gives you power. It fortifies the muscles around your whole midsection and trains them to provide the right amount of support. So if you're weak off the tee, strong abs will improve your distance. But if you also play stop-and-start sports like tennis or squash, strong abs can improve your game tremendously.

The 'Total Body Workout' that begins on page 42 will hit every one of the major muscle groups involved in keeping your core strong and balanced, and the stretches that start every workout will enhance your flexibility and staying power. You'll also notice tips spread throughout the book about how to stay on course, eat the right foods and get the most out of your midsection.

STICK TO THE PROGRAMME

- **Stay positive.** When your brain tells you not to exercise ('The boss is on the warpath, and I'm too stressed to work out'), force a more rational, positive thought into your head: 'Exercise will help me relieve stress. I'll feel worse if I don't exercise this week'. For every negative thought your brain generates, we bet you can counter with three positive ones.

- **Mark off the days.** After you complete a workout, mark down on your calendar what you did that day. If you perform a cardiovascular exercise such as running for 20 minutes, jot down 'C-20'. If you complete your weight-lifting programme, write 'WL'. This gives you written proof of your accomplishments, which studies have shown is strong motivation and reinforcement.

- **Give yourself a reward.** After an especially good workout, treat yourself to a jacuzzi. After a week of consistent exercise, take your girlfriend out for dinner. After a month, buy yourself a CD boxed set. Or come up with your own plan. A long-term study of slightly overweight men showed that self-chosen rewards helped them reach their exercise goals.

- **Join a group or work out with friends.** A review of 113 studies published in the US *Journal of Sport and Exercise Psychology* shows you're more likely to make a lifetime commitment to exercise if you have some kind of social support.

- **While you're exercising, distract yourself from the pain.** Psychologists call this 'disassociation'. You call it television, music or the newspaper. Recent studies suggest that multiple distractions may help you stick to your workout and may even improve your aerobic capacity.

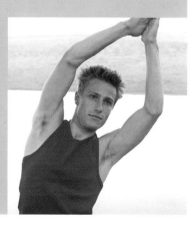

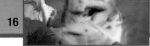

Diet and Nutrition

You're crunching, you're running, you're pounding weights. But if you're not fuelling up and hydrating at the right times with the right food, your six-pack is going to remain in hiding.

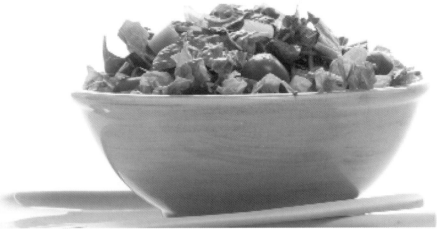

Who says salads can't be manly? Just add hunks of lean beef or chicken for a cool, crunchy meal that's packed with vitamins, fibre, and lean protein.

The Basics

If you want to see your abdominals, you have to get rid of what's hiding them. To do this, you must accomplish two simple dietary goals: eat enough to preserve muscle and don't eat so much that you put on fat. Remember, we said 'simple', not 'easy'. Here are a few basic rules to follow to maintain your midsection:

Fill up with protein and multicoloured vegetables. A high protein diet makes you feel full longer and helps keep your belly flat, whereas eating too many carbohydrates makes you feel bloated. Eat chicken, fish or beef with as many vegetables as you want, the more colourful the better. Orange and yellow peppers, onions, tomatoes, broccoli, spinach and asparagus are all good choices to pair with a protein-rich main course – a steak, chicken breast or tuna steak. Between meals, stick to the protein plan. Snack on hard-boiled eggs or cheese, or make a protein smoothie with soya milk, peanut butter and a banana.

Go easy on 'dry' carbohydrates. After 4 p.m., stay away from carbohy-

ABS-FRIENDLY SMOOTHIE

Pour 2 scoops of vanilla protein powder and 350 ml (12 fl oz) of plain soya milk into a blender. Add a heaped tablespoon of peanut butter, a banana and four ice cubes. If you have some frozen bananas, you can use them instead of the ice cubes. When you go food shopping, buy a lot of bananas at once; as some of them start to turn brown, peel and freeze them to use in shakes. Sprinkle in 4 tbsp of raw oat bran for added fibre. Blend it up and drink it down.

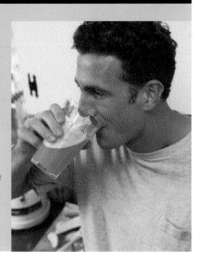

drate-heavy foods that come mostly from grains, or 'dry carbs'. This means no rice, pasta, potatoes or bread in the late afternoon or evening. These foods seem to put flab on the belly. You should still eat a big dinner every night – in addition to a big breakfast, a big lunch and several big snacks. But when the big dinner follows rule number one – tuna with a green salad, for example – you'll wake up in the morning leaner than the day before.

Eat fibre. Fibre keeps you regular and helps your body better assimilate dietary fat. Try sprinkling your cereal with raw oat bran. Start with one tablespoon a day for two weeks, then double that amount. Or cook it porridge-style with raisins and peanut butter; you'll get a lot of fibre, some

protein and healthy fats, all of which will help you feel full much longer than you would by eating, say, cold cereal or a bagel for breakfast.

Consume good fats. Take in approximately 60 to 100 grams of fat per day, from avocados, olive oil, unsalted nuts and peanut butter. A huge mistake some people make: they go fat-free and feel deprived. You must give your body good fats to feel full and satisfied.

One day a week, allow yourself to break every nutrition rule. It's your 'cheat day', and, most important, you should do it without guilt. Be tough on yourself six days a week, and then on the seventh day, take shore leave. Just stick to your healthy diet for the rest of the week. You'll probably find that the day after

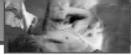

a cheat, you're not very hungry and have no appetite for junk food.

Diet Right

Diets generally fail for one of two reasons: either they're too restrictive about the kind of food you can eat, or they leave you feeling as if you haven't put any food in your belly. In either case, it's usually not long before you have chocolate biscuit crumbs on the corners of your mouth.

You won't be sabotaged by either of those problems with our programme, which was created for us by expert trainers and nutritionists.

If you want to shrink your gut, get enough protein in your diet – about 25 per cent of your daily calories. Why? Protein makes you feel full and helps build muscle (which increases metabolism, thereby making it easier to lose weight). Just as important, high-protein diets have been shown to be the best way to attack belly fat.

Get enough fat – about 30 per cent of your calories each day. First, fat helps you feel fuller longer between meals. Second, it provides essential fatty acids needed for optimal health. Above all, fat makes you feel like you're eating real food, not starving in the land of plenty.

If you get enough protein and fat, your total calorie intake should take care of itself. Because you feel full, you

FAT-BURNING TEA

According to a recent study, men burned more fat when they took a green tea supplement than when they took a caffeine pill or a placebo. And if you drink it iced, four glasses a day can burn more than a kilogram (3 pounds) a year because it takes 30 calories of body heat to warm the tea to 37°C (98.6°F). As for the honey, go easy; studies show that sweeter drinks may stimulate your appetite.

To prepare 3 litres (5 pints) of tea:
Bring 3 litres (5 pints) of water to the boil and then add 4 green tea bags. After a few minutes, stir in 2 tbsp honey. Brew for an hour, remove the tea bags and chill. One glass of tea has 3 calories, 0 g protein, 1 g carbohydrates, 0 g fat and 0 g fibre. It is nice served with fresh mint.

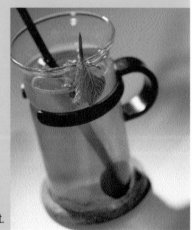

won't binge on a bag of crisps and blow your calorie count for the day. The remaining 45 per cent of calories in our plan comes from carbohydrates – enough to give your palate a full range of tastes and your body a combination of fast and slow burning fuel.

These are all great reasons to pursue an abs-friendly diet. The best reason is this: the programme is an easy, sacrifice-free plan that will let you eat the foods you want and keep you looking and feeling better day after day. It's designed to help you lose weight by recalibrating your body's internal fat-burning furnace. It focuses on foods that trigger your body to start shedding flab, rebuilding you into a lean, mean, fat-burning machine.

YOU MUST EAT FAT

Fat gets a bad rap in many diet plans, but its health benefits are hugely underrated. A diet with 21 per cent of its calories from monounsaturated fat reduces your risk of cardiovascular disease by 25 per cent, according to a recent study. And additional research has shown that men who eat a diet with 40 per cent fat have higher testosterone than those who eat 20 per cent or less. So chomp on those macadamia nuts and drench your salad with olive oil. Not only will you enjoy your food more, you'll live longer and have more sex.

1.5 grams of protein per kilogram of body weight every day is enough to help your body build muscle and burn fat.

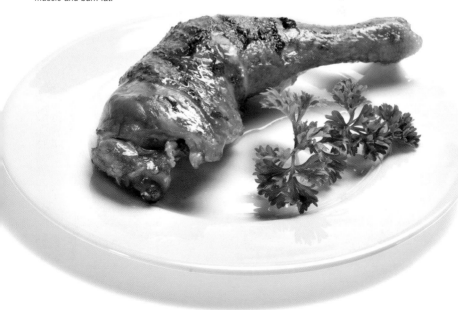

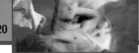

The Abs-Sculpting Diet

The meals shown here are 'templates' that you can modify in any number of ways to keep your tastebuds happy. Follow them and you'll be consuming between 2,400 and 2,800 calories every day. That should provide plenty of calories for all but the most severely obese, while allowing most guys to lose fat from around their middles at a safe and steady pace. (Don't worry about hitting the numbers on the nose every time. If you exceed your fat quota during lunch, for instance, just cut back a bit during dinner.)

TOTAL: 621 kcal, 47 g protein, 50 g carbohydrate, 26 g fat.

Breakfast
- 5 tbsp (40 g) wholegrain flakes or porridge oats
- 150 ml (5 fl oz) skimmed milk
- 2 tbsp chopped nuts
- 2 tbsp raisins

TOTAL: 566 kcal, 20 g protein, 80 g carbohydrate, 19 g fat.

Lunch
- Sandwich made with 2 slices wholemeal bread, 5 oz (150 g) ham or tuna, 1 slice low-fat cheese, 2 slices tomato.
- 1 tbsp mayonnaise
- 1 carrot
- 1 glass (150 ml/5 fl oz) orange juice

Dinner
- 5 oz (150 g) cooked lean meat, poultry or shellfish
- Small green leafy salad
- 2 tsp French dressing

Medium serving (80 g) broccoli
- 4 tbsp (150 g) cooked rice or pasta or potatoes
- 1 medium-sized fruit e.g. apple

TOTAL: 662 kcal, 39 g protein, 60 g carbohydrate, 31 g fat.

Floater Meal
- 2 slices wholemeal bread
- 2 tbsp peanut butter
- 480ml (16 fl oz) skimmed milk
- 1 medium apple

TOTAL: 605 kcal, 32 g protein, 70 g carbohydrate, 23 g fat.

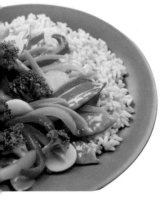

RECIPE KEY
tbsp = tablespoon
tsp = teaspoon

PROTEIN POWER

A study compared high-carbohydrate and high-protein diets for weight loss in extremely overweight men. Even though the number of calories were the same, the high protein group lost 28 per cent more weight in the four-week study. But, more importantly, the metabolic rates of the men in the high protein group were 14 per cent faster than the others. You need no more than 1.5 grams of protein per kilogram of body weight (that's just less than one gram per pound). Any excess will be stored as fat.

If you find it difficult to eat foods that are high in protein, protein supplements are a possible option, but they can be expensive. A single serving of a typical supplement contains between 18 and 40 grams of protein. All are sweetened with a sugar called maltodextrin, so you don't have to add anything but water and then mix them up in a shaker or blender. Two servings can supply your daily protein allowance.

Protein bars are another alternative, with one minor drawback. Many are made with chemicals called sugar alcohols, and too much of these can lead to serious flatulence. But you shouldn't experience this problem with one bar a day.

Sources of Protein

Food	Protein (grams)
170 g can of tuna	39
1 medium (130 g, cooked weight) chicken breast	34
2 thick slices (90 g, cooked weight) lean roast beef	26
roast beef sandwich	22
6 egg whites	18
turkey sandwich on wholemeal bread	18
2 whole eggs	13
small bag (50 g) cashews	10
4 tbsp (160 g) baked beans	8
150 g container low-fat yogurt	8
240 ml skimmed milk	8
small portion (200 g, cooked) spaghetti	7
30 g oatmeal (uncooked)	4

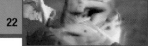

Stretching Basics

Don't make the mistake of diving straight into your abdominal workout. A complete stretching routine can take as little as 10 minutes, and will do wonders for your overall health and fitness. Not only will you decrease the likelihood of pain and soreness after your abs routine, you'll also improve circulation, your range of motion and your ability to relax. Here are some good basic moves that hit all the important areas.

CHEST STRETCH

Try this stretch to work your chest and shoulders. Clasp your hands together, palms up, behind your lower back. Pull your arms up towards your head. Hold for 10 seconds.

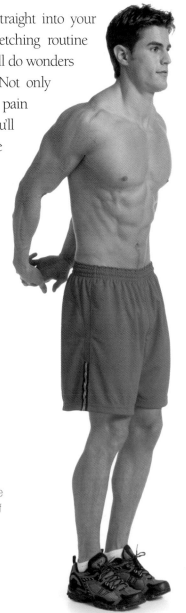

WARM MUSCLES WORK BETTER

When muscles are cold, they're stiff. Light exercise before stretching warms them and makes them more pliable, improving the stretch and reducing the risk of muscle strain. Keep it simple – walk or slowly jog for 10 minutes to prepare your muscles for the exercises ahead.

POSTERIOR SHOULDER STRETCH

Grab the back of your right upper arm with your left hand and pull it across your chest gently. Hold for 10 seconds, and then repeat on the other side.

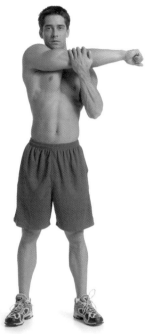

LYING ILIOTIBIAL BAND STRETCH

Lie on your back. Keep your left leg straight and lift it across your body. Hold for 10 seconds. Repeat with the other leg. You will feel this stretch in your hips.

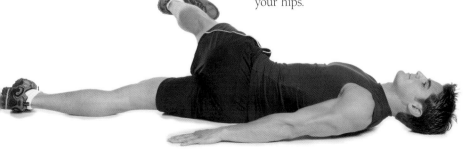

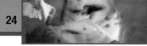

HIP-FLEXOR STRETCH

Plant your left foot on a bench, and then lean towards it, bending your left leg while keeping your right leg straight. Feel the stretch on the front of your right hip. Hold for 30 seconds, and then switch legs.

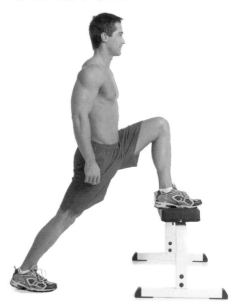

LOWER-BACK STRETCH

This stretch resembles a reclining spread eagle. Lie flat on your stomach. Slowly lift your upper chest, shoulders, neck and head. Make sure you don't strain your neck. As you are doing this, also stretch and lift your lower legs and feet a few centimetres above the ground. Keep your hands behind you and extend them, with fingertips straight out. Stretch from head to toe. Hold for 15 seconds per repetition. Work up to one or two sets of eight repetitions.

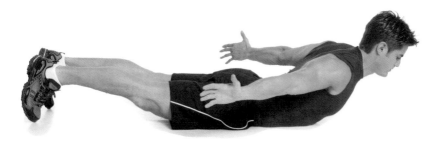

TOWEL STRETCH

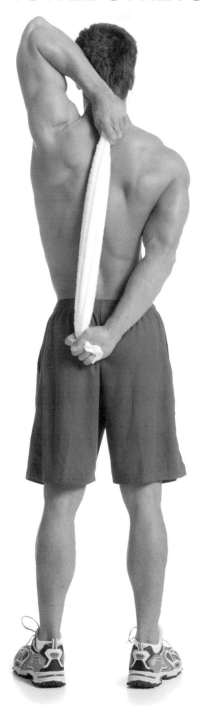

Grab the ends of a towel with your left hand behind your head and your right hand at the middle of your back. Gently pull down with your right hand until you feel a good stretch in your left shoulder and triceps. Hold for 15 to 30 seconds. Then pull up with your left hand until you feel a stretch in your right shoulder, and hold that for 15 to 30 seconds. Repeat two or three times, slowly going from one stretch to the other. Reverse hand positions and repeat two or three more times.

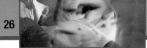

FULL-BODY STRETCH

This is a great stretch to end your workout. Sit on the floor with your left leg straight out in front of you. Bend your right leg and put the sole of your right foot against the inside of your left thigh. (Your legs will look like the number 4.) With your left hand, try to touch either your left ankle or your left big toe. This stretches your left calf, Achilles tendon, hamstring, hip, knee, glutes, lower-back muscles, shoulder and wrist. Hold the position for 30 to 60 seconds, and then switch sides.

DON'T STRETCH TOO FAR

Extend the muscle far enough to make a difference, but not so far that you cause its fibres to tear. Stretch until you feel a slight tug – don't push beyond that point.

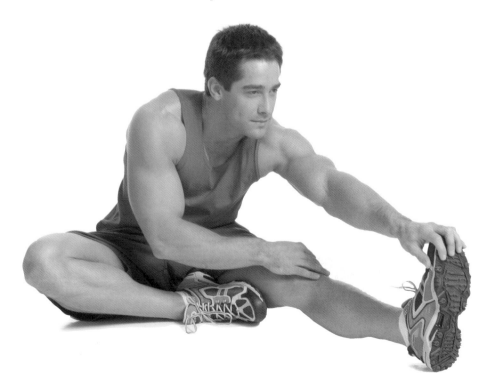

PART II:
Ultimate Workouts

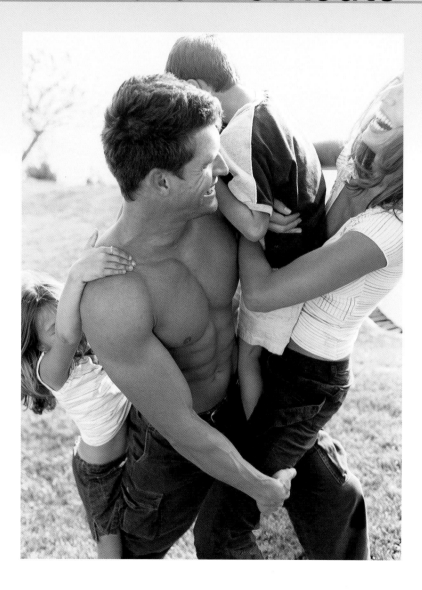

THE 15-MINUTE WORKOUT

Chisel Your Middle

Sucking in your gut doesn't fool anyone – not her, not you, not your tailor. So start using the natural corset you were born with: the *transverse abdominis*. It's the horizontal layer of muscle beneath your six-pack, and it can make your waist thinner.

ROLLBACK

Targets: Transverse Abdominis
Time: 5 Minutes

1 Sit with your knees bent and your heels on the floor. Keep your torso upright, shoulders back and arms extended forwards, parallel to the floor. Inhale while keeping your belly pulled in.

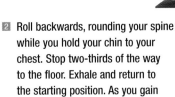

2 Roll backwards, rounding your spine while you hold your chin to your chest. Stop two-thirds of the way to the floor. Exhale and return to the starting position. As you gain strength, roll back closer to the floor.

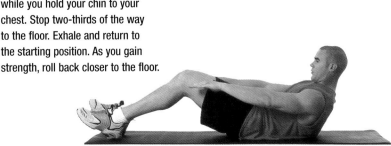

TOE TAP

Targets: Rectus Abdominis, Transverse Abdominis
Time: 5 Minutes

1. Lie on your back and place your fingers behind your ears. Lift your left leg until the lower leg is parallel to the floor. Press your lower back against the floor and crunch forwards until your shoulders are off the floor.

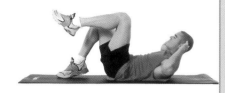

2. With your toes pointed down, lower your left foot as far as you can without lifting your back off the floor (not pictured). Return to the starting position and repeat with your right leg.

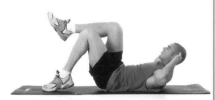

LEG LIFT PRESS-UP

Targets: Obliques, Transverse Abdominis, Spinal Erectors, Gluteals, Chest, Shoulders, Triceps
Time: 5 Minutes

1. Get into the down position of a press-up, your hands in line with your shoulders, about 15 centimetres away from your body. Place your feet hip-width apart. Push up by straightening your arms. Then raise your right leg as high as you can.

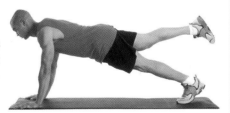

2. Keeping your leg raised, perform a normal press-up by lowering your chest to the floor. Keep your back flat and your body rigid. Switch legs on each repetition.

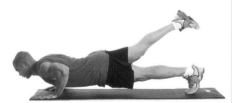

TRAINER'S TIP

If the Leg Lift Press-up is too tough, try it without the press-up. Get into press-up position, and tighten your midsection so your back is perfectly flat – a straight line from neck to ankles. Now lift one leg slowly, pause, lower it slowly and repeat with the other.

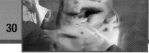

Carve Your Abs

Get Beach-Ready Abs in 3 Weeks

When the thought of a day at the beach keeps you up at night – and your fears have nothing to do with shark attacks or melanoma – it's time to skim the fat once and for all. Try this 3-week total body workout from the strength coach Ian King.

Frequency

Do each workout (Day 1, Day 2 and Day 3) once a week for 3 weeks, then rest a week.

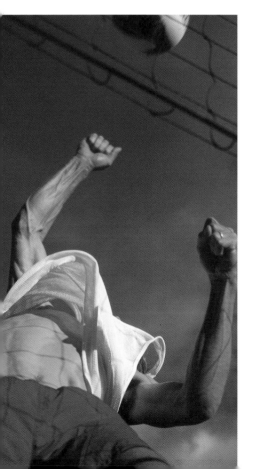

Abdominal Routines

You'll do the same five abdominal exercises during each workout:

- **Day 1–Control:** On each rep, take 3 seconds to lift your body, pause, then lower for 3 seconds.
- **Day 2–Power:** Use light weights; lift your body as fast as you can, and lower in 1 second (no pause).
- **Day 3–Endurance:** Take 2 seconds to raise your body and 1 second to lower it (no pause).

Circuit Sets

Do the exercises in the order they appear in the workout charts on pages 31–32 as circuit sets, that is, one after another without rest. When you use weights, circuits can be a great total body workout. But they're most valuable without weights as a warm-up of the nervous system, joints and muscles.

You'll jump higher and punch better on the volleyball court if you develop your *rectus abdominis* – the six-pack muscle.

ABS ROUTINE: Control	DAY 1	BEGINNER REPS	ADVANCED REPS
	Reverse crunch (p.55)	10–15	10–15
	Situp (p.70)	10–15	10–15
	Russian twist (p.71)	10–15	10–15
	Toe touch (p.72)	10–15	10–15
	Modified V-sit (p.73)	10–15	10–15
TOTAL BODY	Aerobic Station		
	Jump squat (p.88)	10–15	8–12
	Aerobic Station		
	Lat pull-down (p.86)	10–15	8–12
	Aerobic Station		
	Jump shrug (p.88)	10–15	8–12
	Aerobic Station		
	Shoulder press (p.81)	10–15	8–12
	Aerobic Station		

ABS ROUTINE: Power	DAY 2	BEGINNER REPS	ADVANCED REPS
	Reverse crunch (p.55)	10–15	10–15
	Situp (p.70)	10–15	10–15
	Russian twist (p.71)	10–15	10–15
	Toe touch (p.72)	10–15	10–15
	Modified V-sit (p.73)	10–15	10–15
TOTAL BODY	Aerobic Station		
	Walking lunge (p.90)	10–15	8–12
	Aerobic Station		
	Dips (p.82)	10–15	8–12
	Aerobic Station		
	Windmill lunge (p.91)	5/leg	5/leg
	Aerobic Station		
	Lat pull-down (p.86)	10–15	8–12
	Aerobic Station		

DAY 3		BEGINNER REPS	ADVANCED REPS
ABS ROUTINE: Endurance	Reverse crunch (p.55)	10–15	15–20
	Situp (p.70)	10–15	15–20
	Russian twist (p.71)	10–15	15–20
	Toe touch (p.72)	10–15	15–20
	Modified V-sit (p.73)	10–15	15–20
TOTAL BODY	Aerobic Station		
	Power clean and press (p.83)	10–15	8–12
	Aerobic Station		
	Bench press (p.80)	10–15	8–12
	Aerobic Station		
	Barbell squat (p.89)	10–15	8–12
	Aerobic Station		
	Barbell bent-over row (p.84)	10–15	8–12
	Aerobic Station		

- **Week 1**–Do one circuit (one set of each exercise).
- **Week 2**–Do two circuits (two sets of each exercise).
- **Week 3**–Do three circuits (three sets of each exercise).

Speed of Repetitions

Take 1 second to lower the weight, then without pausing, lift the weight as quickly as you can. Even though you're using the weights explosively in this workout, maintain control over them through all stages of the lift. Always maintain a firm grip on the bar or dumbbell, and make sure you use weight (grip) collars.

Aerobic Stations

You'll do these cardio activities in between the exercises that follow the abs routine. Start with 30 seconds of any continuous-motion exercise you choose. You can jog around an indoor track, if your gym has one; hop on any piece of cardiovascular equipment you have access to; or do something as simple as jumping jacks, shadow boxing, skipping or running on the spot.

Add 15 seconds to your aerobic stations each time you do a

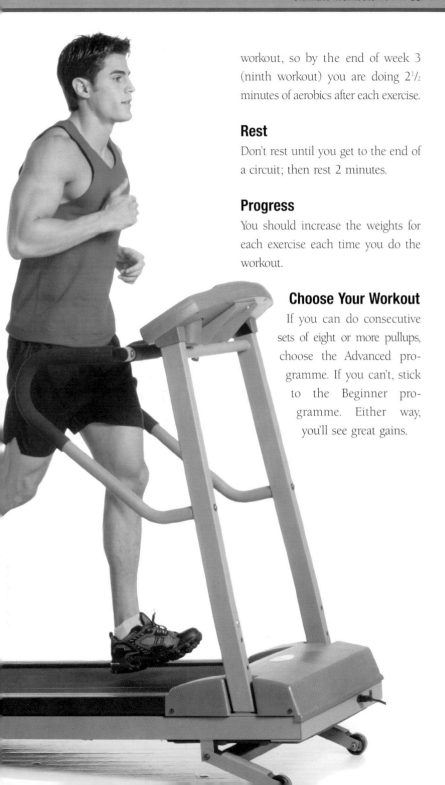

workout, so by the end of week 3 (ninth workout) you are doing 2½ minutes of aerobics after each exercise.

Rest

Don't rest until you get to the end of a circuit; then rest 2 minutes.

Progress

You should increase the weights for each exercise each time you do the workout.

Choose Your Workout

If you can do consecutive sets of eight or more pullups, choose the Advanced programme. If you can't, stick to the Beginner programme. Either way, you'll see great gains.

Abs in No Time

Grab a medicine ball for an intensified crunch workout that will flatten your belly before the summer holiday season. These state of the art exercises use the weight of a medicine ball to blast your belly from top to bottom, and your obliques on the sides – those all-important muscles you use when doing twisting, turning moves in sports. The added weight of the medicine ball will give you a more intense workout than you'll get with conventional crunches. If a weighted ball is too challenging (or if you're doing this at home and don't have one), try the workout using a basket-ball, football or volleyball. Start these core exercises now, it's never too early – or too late – to chisel beach-ready abs.

Work your abs standing up and they'll do double duty, stabilizing the spine and keeping you upright.

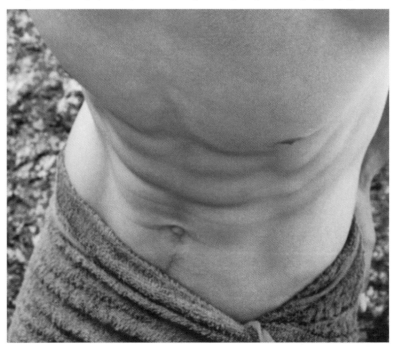

DOUBLE CRUNCH

Targets: Rectus Abdominis, Obliques, Inner Thighs

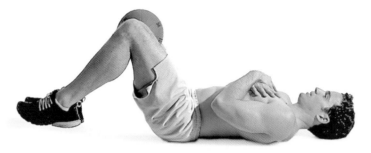

1 Lie on your back, with your hips and knees bent as shown and your feet off the floor. Rest your hands lightly on your chest. Position the ball between your knees.

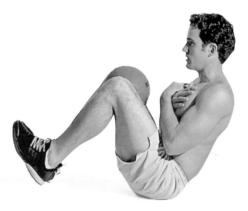

2 Exhale as you lift your shoulders off the floor and bring your knees towards your chest.

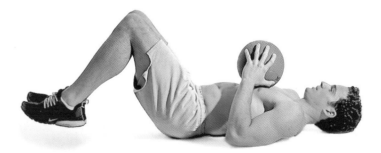

3 Grab the ball with your hands and bring it to your chest as you inhale and return your shoulders and legs to the starting position. Transfer the ball back to your legs on the next repetition, and keep alternating ball positions for the entire set.

SEATED TWIST

Targets: Obliques

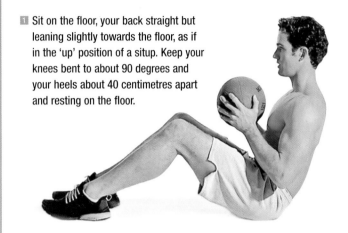

1 Sit on the floor, your back straight but leaning slightly towards the floor, as if in the 'up' position of a situp. Keep your knees bent to about 90 degrees and your heels about 40 centimetres apart and resting on the floor.

2 Hold the ball close to your chest, rotate your torso to the left and place the ball on the floor behind you.

3 Rotate around to the right, pick up the ball, rotate left and place it behind you.

4 Repeat eight to 12 times, then do eight to 12 more starting with a rotation to your right; that's one set.

TRAINER'S TIP

Keep your head in line with your torso throughout the movement. Perform this move as quickly as possible.

REVERSE CRUNCH WITH KNEE DROPS

Targets: Rectus Abdominis, Obliques, Hip Flexors

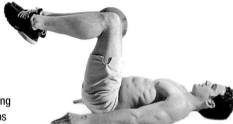

1. Lie on your back, hands resting on the floor at your sides, hips and knees bent 90 degrees, and feet off the floor. Position the ball between your knees. Keep your lower back on the floor throughout the exercise.

2. Contract your abdominals and pull your knees to your chest, then return them to the starting position.

3. Lower your knees to the left and return to the starting position. Drop your knees to your right on the next repetition, and alternate sides for each rep.

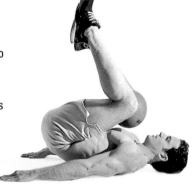

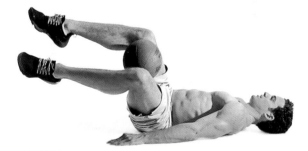

CHOOSE YOUR BALL

Use a ball that's light enough so you can do one set of each exercise without straining or arching your back. A good weight for ab workouts is about 4 kilograms.

Start with one circuit and build up to three sets of the circuit. Use a slow, controlled movement for the double crunch and reverse crunch.

8-Week Belly-Off Programme

Lost your abs? Well, the good news is they're not gone. The bad news – they're hiding under layers of fat that have settled around your middle. If you're serious about shedding those layers, this programme is designed with you in mind. It includes rigorous upper and lower body weight-lifting workouts, an aerobic routine, an interval workout *and* the Belly-Off routine. Here's all you need to know and what you need to *do* to get your body back:

Belly-Off Routine

To finally reveal those hidden abs, do these exercises twice a week, for 8 weeks. You can perform this 15-minute routine in two ways:

- Do three sets of each exercise. Rest 30 to 60 seconds between sets and before moving on to the next exercise.
- Do all five exercises as a circuit without rest between individual exercises. Do three circuits, resting 1 to 2 minutes in between.

Upper-Body Workout

Do these exercises in pairs as super-sets – one straight after the other, no rest. Rest 30 to 60 seconds between supersets, and do each superset three times. Perform this workout twice a week for 8 weeks.

Lower-Body Workout

Do all five leg exercises, plus the clams, as one set with no breaks. Rest 1½ to 2 minutes after the ordeal, and repeat twice more. Do this workout twice a week for 8 weeks.

Aerobic Routine

Twice a week, do 20 to 30 minutes of steady, medium-intensity cardio-vascular exercise after weight work-outs. Increase the cardio sessions by 5 minutes every 2 weeks.

Interval Workout

Twice a week, on days you don't lift weights, warm up for 5 minutes, then go hard at it for 30 seconds, easy for 1½ to 2 minutes and repeat for a total of 10 to 12 intervals. Cool down for 5 minutes.

Belly-Off Routine

EXERCISE	REPS
Hanging leg raise (p.78)	6–10
Swiss ball jackknife (p.57)	6–8
Oblique crunch (each side, p.58)	10–12
Cable crunch (p.62)	8–12
Swiss ball bridge (p.76)	hold 15–30 secs

Upper-Body Workout

	EXERCISE	REPS
SET 1	Bench press (p.80)	8–10
	Cable row (p.85)	10–12
SET 2	Lat pull-down (p.86)	10–12
	Shoulder press (p.81)	10–12
SET 3	Dips (p.82)	8–10
	Dumbbell upright row (p.84)	10–12
SET 4	Reverse crunch (p.55)	12–15
	Back extension (p.94)	10–12

Lower-Body Workout

EXERCISE	REPS
Barbell squat (p.89)	10–12
Leg extension (p.93)	12–15
Dumbbell stepup (each leg, p.87)	10–12
Lying leg curl (p.92)	10–12
Calf raise (p.93)	10–12
Clam (p.59)	12–15

THE 15-MINUTE WORKOUT

A Stronger Core

With this unique circuit, you'll lunge, twist and swing your way to powerful core muscles. These moves will help you develop total body strength, stability and flexibility, reducing your risk of suffering many common sports-related injuries, including twisted knees and pulled shoulders. Perform this workout 2 or 3 days a week, resting for at least 1 day between sessions. Do the exercises one after another in circuit fashion, resting 15 seconds after each exercise. When you've completed one set of each, rest 1 minute, then repeat the sequence two more times.

TWISTING SHOULDER PRESS

Targets: Deltoids, Trapezius, Obliques

1 Hold dumbbells outside your shoulders at jaw level, palms facing in. Press the dumbbells overhead as you twist your torso to the left.

2 Lower the dumbbells as you twist back to the centre, then press upwards again while twisting to the right. Do six repetitions in each direction.

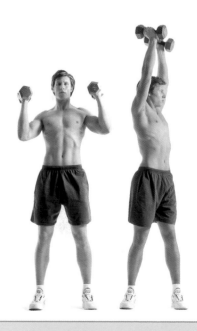

DUMBBELL SWING

Targets: Gluteals, Hamstrings, Lower Back, Deltoids

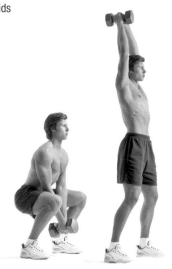

1. Stand holding a dumbbell with a hand-over-hand grip at arm's length in front of your waist. Bend at your knees and waist (keep your back flat) until your upper body is about 45 degrees from vertical and the dumbbell is between your knees.

2. Swing the dumbbell up and directly over your head (as if you were lifting an axe) as you straighten your knees and back and push your hips forwards.

3. Pause, then lower the dumbbell back to the starting position and repeat. Do eight repetitions.

OVERHEAD LUNGE

Targets: Whole Lower Body, Shoulders, Obliques

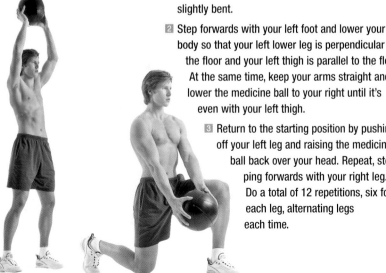

1. Hold a medicine ball at arm's length over your head, your feet hip-width apart and your knees slightly bent.

2. Step forwards with your left foot and lower your body so that your left lower leg is perpendicular to the floor and your left thigh is parallel to the floor. At the same time, keep your arms straight and lower the medicine ball to your right until it's even with your left thigh.

3. Return to the starting position by pushing off your left leg and raising the medicine ball back over your head. Repeat, stepping forwards with your right leg. Do a total of 12 repetitions, six for each leg, alternating legs each time.

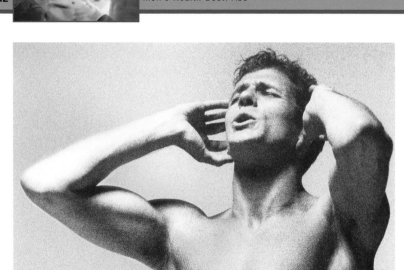

With the right combination of diet and exercise, you'll begin to discover muscles you never knew existed.

Total Body
Workout

This 8-week abs-building programme works your whole midsection – not just the six-pack muscle (*rectus abdominis*), but also your obliques and lower back. Some of the exercises even strengthen the deep abdominal and lower-back muscles that help you sit up straighter when you aren't moving.

Beginner Workout

	EXERCISE	WEEKS 1–2 REPS	WEEKS 3–4 REPS	WEEKS 5–6 REPS	WEEKS 7–8 REPS
ABDOMINAL ROUTINE	Bridge (p.74)	2	2	–	–
	Russian twist (p.71)	10–12	12–15	–	–
	Towel crunch (p.60)	10–12	12–15	–	–
	Back extension (p.94)	10–12	12–15	–	–
	Two-point bridge (p.74)	–	–	4–6	6–8
	Hanging leg raise (p.78)	–	–	4–6	6–8
	Reverse woodchopper (p.67)	–	–	4–6	6–8
	Swiss ball crunch (p.52)	–	–	4–6	6–8
TOTAL BODY ROUTINE	Lat pull-down (p.86)	8–12	8–12	8–12	8–12
	Barbell squat (p.89)	8–12	8–12	8–12	8–12
	Lying leg curl (p.92)	8–12	8–12	8–12	8–12
	Bench press (p.80)	8–12	8–12	8–12	8–12
	Cable row (p.85)	8–12	8–12	8–12	8–12
	Lying triceps extension (p.82)	8–12	8–12	8–12	8–12
	Biceps curl (p.81)	8–12	8–12	8–12	8–12

Beginner Workout

If you're new to weight lifting or are returning to it after a long break, choose this workout. Do your abs exercises followed by the total body routine two or three times a week.

- **Abdominal Routine:** Do 2 sets of each exercise during Weeks 1–2 and Weeks 5–6. Do 2–3 sets of each exercise during Weeks 3–4 and Weeks 7–8. (See above workout chart for exercise repetitions.)

- **Total Body Routine:** Do 1 set of each exercise for all 8 weeks of the programme. The exercises listed in the chart are just suggestions.

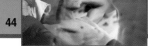

Intermediate Workout

Choose this workout *if* you:

- have been lifting weights for at least 6 months to a year
- have tried several different workout programmes
- have seen improvements in strength and muscle mass

Divide your programme into two workouts, one for your upper body and one for your lower body. Perform your abdominal exercises on the day you do your lower-body workout. Alternate between the two workouts, taking a day off after each.

- **Abdominal Routine:** Do 2 sets of each exercise during Weeks 1–2 and Weeks 5–6. Do 2–3 sets of each exercise during Weeks 3–4 and Weeks 7–8.
- **Upper-Body Workout:** Do two or three sets of the chest and back exercises and one or two sets of the exercises for the arms.
- **Lower-Body Workout:** After doing the abdominal routine, do two or three warmup sets and two work sets of both these moves. (A work set means you're using the most weight you can for that number of repetitions. The warmup sets should be percentages of that weight – maybe 40, 60 and 80 per cent. Do fewer repetitions in each warmup set.)

Stretching Essentials

Don't dive straight into your weight-training workout – stretch before you train, and warm up before you stretch. Do about 10 minutes of low-intensity work on an exercise bike or a treadmill to decrease the chance of injury and to elevate your body temperature before performing strenuous or demanding exercises. Once your muscles are warm, stretch them for another 5 to 10 minutes, focusing on the body parts you plan to train.

You can help prevent muscle soreness after your workout by cooling down with light aerobic exercise for about 5 minutes and then stretching for another 5 to 10 minutes. You can use the stretches on pages 22–26 to warm up before you train, or to cool down after your workout.

Aerobic Training

Do 20 to 30 minutes of your favourite cardiovascular exercise – jogging, rowing, cycling – twice a week. Perform your cardio routine after your lifting session, during another part of the day, or better still, on a day when you aren't working with weights. If possible, avoid aerobic exercise before your lifting sessions – this causes your muscles to fatigue and you'll burn out before you get to the weight training.

Intermediate Workout

	EXERCISE	WEEKS 1–2 REPS	WEEKS 3–4 REPS	WEEKS 5–6 REPS	WEEKS 7–8 REPS
ABS ROUTINE	Two-point bridge (p.74)	4–6	6–8	–	–
	Hanging leg raise (p.78)	4–6	6–8	–	–
	Reverse woodchopper (p.67)	4–6	6–8	–	–
	Swiss ball crunch (p.52)	4–6	6–8	–	–
	Swiss ball jackknife (p.57)	–	–	3–5	5–8
	Oblique hanging leg raise (p.79)	–	–	3–5	5–8
	Twisting back extension (p.94)	–	–	3–5	5–8
	Swiss ball circle crunch (p.53)	–	–	3–5	5–8
TOTAL BODY ROUTINE	Dumbbell stepup (p.87)	8–12	8–12	8–12	8–12
	Barbell squat (p.89) or Walking lunge (p.90)	8–12	8–12	8–12	8–12
	Calf raise (p.93)	8–12	8–12	8–12	8–12
	Bench press (p.80)	8–12	8–12	8–12	8–12
	Lat pull-down (p.86)	8–12	8–12	8–12	8–12
	Biceps curl (p.81)	8–12	8–12	8–12	8–12
	Lying triceps extension (p.82)	8–12	8–12	8–12	8–12

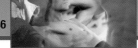

Isolate Your Abs

6 Moves for a Perfect, Powerful Midsection

If you've been diligently working your midsection but remain a few cans short of a six-pack, there may be a simple explanation. You need the right diet and exercise programme (weights and cardiovascular) to burn fat before you can develop a washboard stomach. But even before you whittle down that fatty layer, you should condition your abdominal muscles with a few good moves that isolate your midsection. Perform the abdominal routine at the beginning of your workout.

Abs Isolation Workout

Choose one of the abs exercises from each row of the exercise grid on the following page and perform the number of reps and sets recommended for your fitness level. For each repetition, take 3–4 seconds to curl up, and 3–4 seconds to return smoothly to the starting position. Whichever moves you choose, you'll hit your abs from several angles to build a strong, flat midsection.

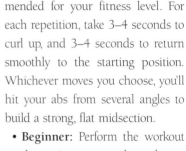

- **Beginner:** Perform the workout three times a week and rest 30–60 seconds between sets.
- **Intermediate:** Perform the workout twice a week and rest 60–90 seconds between sets.
- **Advanced:** Perform the workout twice a week and rest 90–240 seconds between sets. If the exercises aren't challenging enough for you, use weight plates or medicine balls to add resistance.

Attack the excess layers around your middle with at least 20 minutes of aerobic exercise three times a week.

MANAGE YOUR MIDDLE

We talk about six-packs, but the real number is four – your abdominal muscles are divided into four distinct groups. The six exercises in this workout hit them all, while giving you enough variety to keep things interesting. Here's a breakdown of the exercises and the muscles they target.

- Crunch: rectus abdominis
- Weighted crunch: whole rectus abdominis
- Cable crunch: upper rectus abdominis, obliques
- Twisting legs-up crunch: upper and lower rectus abdominis, obliques
- Twisting crunch: upper and lower rectus abdominis, obliques
- Swiss ball stability pose: transverse abdominis isolation

EXERCISE	REPS	BEGINNER SETS	INTERMEDIATE SETS	ADVANCED SETS
Crunch (p.50)	10–15	2–3	2–4	3–5
Weighted crunch (p.63), Cable crunch (p.62) or Pulse twist (p.65)	10–15	2–3	2–4	3–5
Twisting legs-up crunch (p.64) or Twisting crunch (p.51)	10–15	2–3	2–4	3–5
Swiss ball stability pose (p.77)	10–15	2–3	2–4	3–5

Don't Waste Your Workout

What you do before, during and after a workout can either negate your hard work or elevate your growth. Here are a few common saboteurs.

- **Don't skip the basics.** Contrary to popular belief, doing isolation exercises like chest flies and leg extensions is not the only way to increase muscle. Basic moves such as bench presses (page 80) and squats (pages 88 and 89) force several muscle groups to work together, imposing more stress on your body for bigger gains. For maximum results, at least 40 to 50 per cent of your workout should consist of compound moves.

- **Don't play too hard.** Playing sports too often can sidetrack your muscle-growth goals. Muscles typically need 48 hours of rest to adapt to the stresses placed on them during exercise. Pull your cardiovascular activity back to the bare minimum – 20 minutes, three times a week – to see how it affects your body. If cardio is indeed stealing your muscle, you should begin to notice strength improvements – being able to lift more weight or complete more repetitions – within 2 to 3 weeks. If your primary goal is to increase muscle, try pulling back further.

- **Stop smoking.** Smoking puts carbon monoxide in your system, which prevents your muscles from getting the oxygen they use for energy. Less oxygen means less efficient muscle contractions and a limited capacity for work.

- **Don't get drunk.** Regular drinking can lower your testosterone levels, decrease overall muscle mass and cover your abs with a layer of fat that interferes with muscle-building hormones. However, drinking moderately (two drinks or fewer per day) won't harm testosterone levels and can actually improve your cardiovascular health.

- **Eat enough.** Straight after a session, your body hurries to convert glucose into glycogen so your muscles can repair themselves and grow. If you don't eat after exercise, your body breaks down muscle into amino acids to convert into glucose. After you work out, eat a high-carbohydrate meal – and don't forget the protein.

- **Sleep enough.** When you work out on insufficient sleep, you exercise at a lower intensity than you realize – but you feel as if it's high. So your muscles are less likely to receive enough stress to grow. Go to bed and wake up at set times every day, even at weekends, to keep your sleep cycles regular.

PART III:
The Exercises

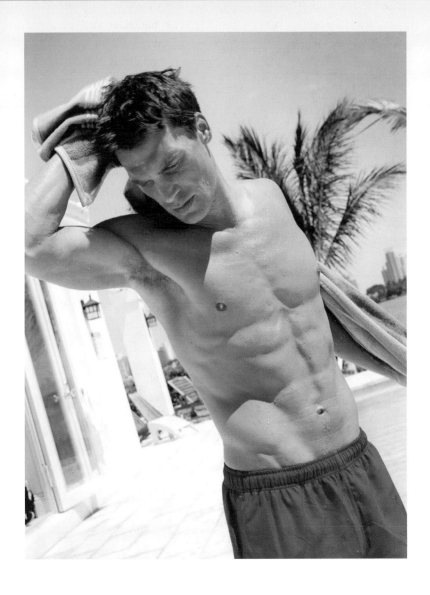

Crunch

The most popular abdominal exercise – the crunch – remains one of the best ways to sculpt an amazing midsection. A well-done crunch is a thing of beauty. Feet flat on the floor, hands behind the ears, slow and steady movements up and down. Nothing rushed, no movement wasted. Although the traditional crunch relies mostly on the upper part of your *rectus abdominis* – the six-pack muscle – there are countless variations that target other key abdominal muscles, including the *transverse abdominis*, the internal and external obliques. So flick through the following pages, take a quick look at your new arsenal of abs-busting exercise and hit the mat!

CRUNCH

Targets: Rectus Abdominis, Obliques

1. Lie on your back with your knees and hips bent about 90 degrees, and cross your arms.
2. Raise your upper body off the floor by crunching your ribcage towards your pelvis. Then lower yourself to the starting position.

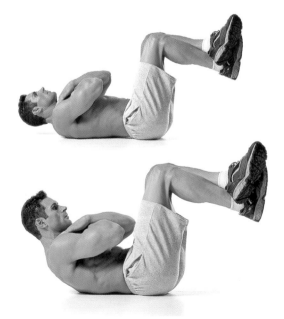

TWISTING CRUNCH

Targets: Upper and Lower Rectus Abdominis, Obliques

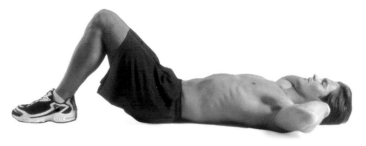

■ Lie on your back with your legs bent at 90 degrees and your feet on the floor. Touch your hands lightly to the sides of your head.

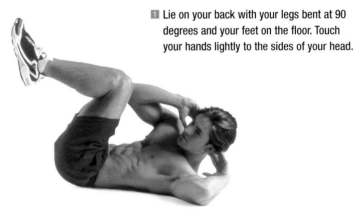

② Slowly lift your shoulders off the ground and twist your body to the left so your right elbow points between your knees. At the same time, draw your knees up and in to meet the elbow.

③ Lower yourself back down and repeat the move, this time twisting to the right so that your left elbow points between your knees.

TRAINER'S TIP

Where you place your hands can change the degree of difficulty of a crunch. If you can't complete the last repetition of a set, try moving your hands from behind your ears to across your chest. This displaces a portion of your weight and may allow you to do one or two more crunches, to work the muscles a bit longer.

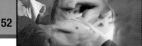

SWISS BALL CRUNCH

■ **Targets:** Obliques, Rectus Abdominis

1 Lie on your back on the ball with your feet flat on the floor. Lower your head as far as you can. Hold your hands behind your ears.

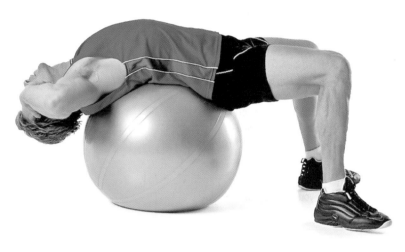

2 Use your abdominal muscles to pull your torso to a sitting position. Pause, then slowly lower yourself.

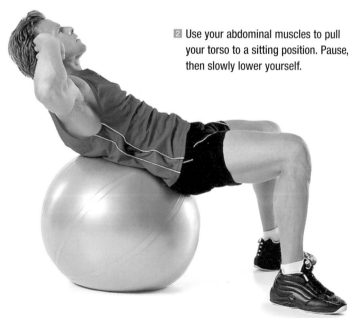

SWISS BALL CIRCLE CRUNCH

■ **Targets:** Rectus Abdominis, Obliques

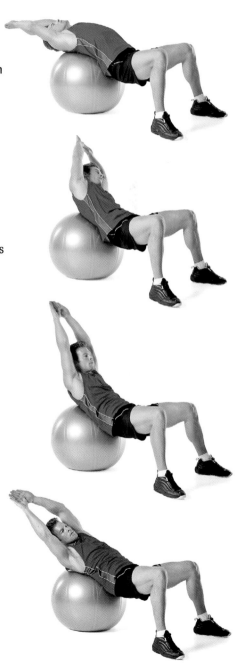

1. Lie on your back on a Swiss ball with your arms extended straight above your head – in line with your ears – and your thumbs crossed so that they interlock.

2. Raise your head and shoulders and crunch your ribcage towards your right hip, then continue contracting your abdominals to move your torso anti-clockwise until you're crunching upwards, then left, then down, so that your upper body moves in a circle.

3. Each circle you complete is one repetition.

THE SWISS BALL BENEFIT

Positioning your head, shoulders and back on the ball forces your muscles to contract before you begin the crunch. It also allows you to work your abs through a greater range of motion without compromising your spine.

SWISS BALL REVERSE CRUNCH

■ **Targets:** Obliques, Rectus Abdominis, Hip Flexors

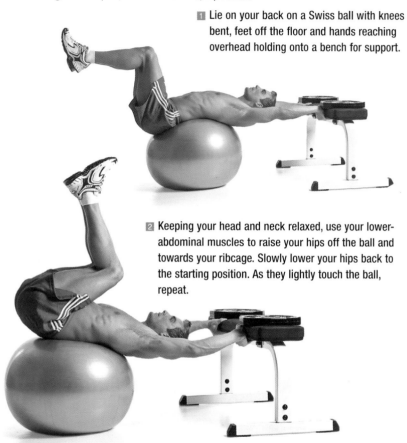

1 Lie on your back on a Swiss ball with knees bent, feet off the floor and hands reaching overhead holding onto a bench for support.

2 Keeping your head and neck relaxed, use your lower-abdominal muscles to raise your hips off the ball and towards your ribcage. Slowly lower your hips back to the starting position. As they lightly touch the ball, repeat.

HOW'S YOUR CRUNCH?
Fix poor form before it becomes a habit

MISTAKE: You pull your head forwards when you crunch, instead of keeping it in line with your body. This makes the exercise less effective, and it can hurt your neck.

FIX: Place your fingers behind your ears or at your temples instead of locking them behind your head, and imagine there's a tennis ball underneath your chin that prevents you from pressing your chin to your chest.

REVERSE CRUNCH

■ **Targets:** Rectus Abdominis, Hip Flexors

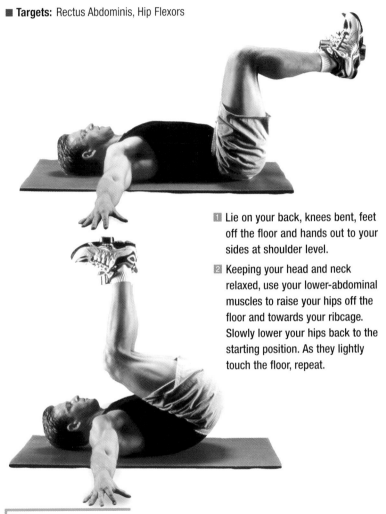

1. Lie on your back, knees bent, feet off the floor and hands out to your sides at shoulder level.

2. Keeping your head and neck relaxed, use your lower-abdominal muscles to raise your hips off the floor and towards your ribcage. Slowly lower your hips back to the starting position. As they lightly touch the floor, repeat.

TRAINER'S TIPS

- Don't quickly rock up and down. You'd be using momentum to aid you in the exercise, taking work away from your lower abs.

- Keep constant tension on your abs – don't rest between repetitions.

- Use your hands for balance. Don't use them to push your hips off the floor.

- For a more challenging exercise, hold a light dumbbell or medicine ball between your ankles.

Jackknife

Most guys think of their abs as one continuous slab of muscle, so they do one continuous set of exercises: crunches. If you really want to etch an impressive midsection though, it's better to think of your abs as having two distinct sections. Crunches are fine for the top half, but to define what's below the waistband, you need exercises that focus on the hip flexors and the lower half of the *rectus abdominis*. Add these moves to your workout routine to develop an even tighter, stronger and leaner middle.

SEATED JACKKNIFE

Targets: Rectus Abdominis, Hip Flexors, Obliques

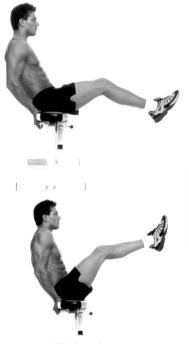

1 Sit on the edge of a sturdy chair or bench, holding the seat behind you for support. Extend your legs in front of you, knees slightly bent.

2 Now, simultaneously raise your legs towards your chest and bring your chest towards your knees.

TRAINER'S TIPS

• Do this exercise at the end of your workout, when your muscles are thoroughly warm, and make sure you stretch your hamstrings between sets. The more limber these muscles are, the harder you'll be able to work your abdominals.

• Try to perform three sets of as many repetitions as you can manage.

SWISS BALL PRESS-UP/JACKKNIFE

Targets: Rectus Abdominis, Hip Flexors, Obliques, Chest, Front Shoulders, Triceps

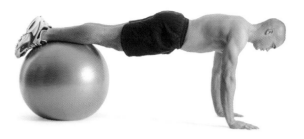

1 Get into press-up position – your hands set slightly wider than and in line with your shoulders – but instead of placing your feet on the floor, rest your shins on a Swiss ball. With your arms straight and your back flat, your body should form a straight line from your shoulders to your ankles.

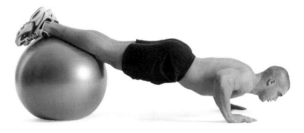

2 Lower your body until your chest nearly touches the floor. Pause, then push yourself back up to the starting position.

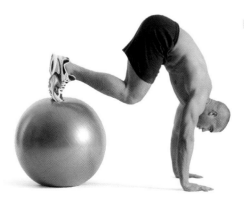

3 Now, roll the Swiss ball towards your chest by raising your hips and rounding your back as you pull the ball forwards with your feet. Pause, then roll the ball back to the starting position. That's one repetition.

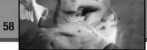

OBLIQUE CRUNCH

■ **Targets:** Obliques

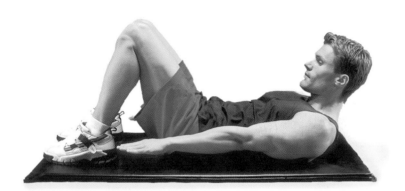

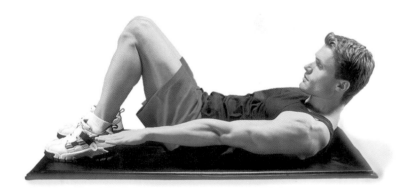

1 Lie on your back with your knees bent, your feet flat on the floor and your arms straight at your sides. Raise your head and shoulders off the floor, into a crunch position.

2 Now reach with your left hand towards your left foot. Return to the crunch position, and reach with your right. That's one repetition.

CLAM

■ **Targets:** Obliques

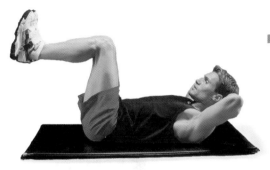

1 Lie on your back with your hips and knees bent 90 degrees so your thighs are perpendicular to your torso and your lower legs are parallel to the floor. Place your hands behind your head with your elbows straight out to your sides.

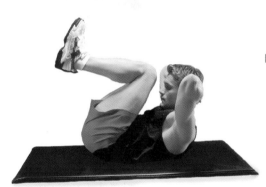

2 Lift your head and shoulders off the floor, like a standard crunch, and at the same time lift your hips off your floor, crunching your knees up towards your chest.

THE SCIENCE OF A POWERFUL CRUNCH

Remember physics? Neither do we. But physics makes the weighted crunch – a great ab chiseller – even better. 'To make your abs work equally hard during both phases of the exercise, extend the weight above your head as you lower your body,' says professional fitness consultant John Paul Catanzaro. For the best results, choose a weight you can crunch six times at the most.

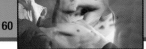

TOWEL CRUNCH

■ **Targets:** Rectus Abdominis, Transverse Abdominis

Space your feet about hip-width apart and plant them firmly on the floor.

Keep your abs in a constant state of contraction through-out the exercise to strengthen your *transverse abdominis*.

Place your fingers lightly behind your ears or cross them on your chest.

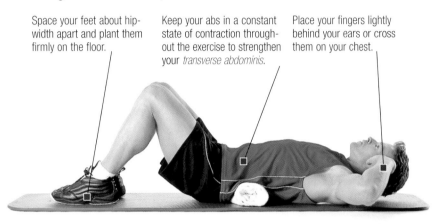

Your tailbone and lower back should stay in contact with the floor throughout the exercise.

Try not to roll your shoulders up and forwards. This places strain on the upper back and neck while making the crunch easier – and less effective.

Keep your head in alignment with your spine and your eyes looking up.

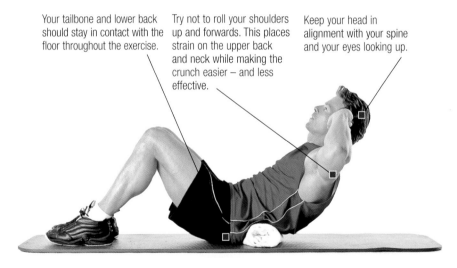

1 Lie on your back with your knees bent and feet flat on the floor spread about hip-width apart. Fold your arms across your chest or place your hands so that they're lightly touching your head behind your ears – but don't pull on your neck. Set a rolled-up towel under the arch of your lower back and lie back so your head rests on the floor.

2 As you begin to exhale, slowly curl your head and torso towards your knees until your shoulder blades are off the floor. Use your upper abs to raise your ribcage towards your pelvis.

3 Hold for a few seconds, then slowly return to the starting position using a controlled motion.

SICILIAN CRUNCH

■ **Targets:** Rectus Abdominis, Transverse Abdominis

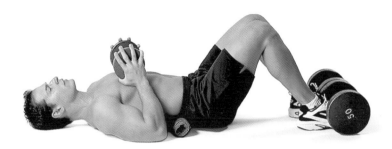

1. Slide your feet under the handles of heavy dumbbells. Place a rolled-up towel under your lower back and hold a dumbbell across your upper chest.

2. Raise your upper body as high as possible by crunching your ribcage towards your pelvis. At the top of the move, straighten your arms and raise the dumbbell above your head.

3. Keep the dumbbell above your head and take 4 seconds to lower your body to the starting position.

TRAINER'S TIPS

On page 7, we said to avoid situps with anchored feet. But we like this exercise because the most important part is when you're lowering your body. Having your feet anchored won't activate your hip flexors to the same degree.

When you don't have time to spare for a complete workout, try doing a quick circuit of Sicilian Crunches. Do five sets of four to six reps, resting 3 minutes after each set.

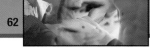

CABLE CRUNCH

■ **Targets:** Rectus Abdominis, Obliques

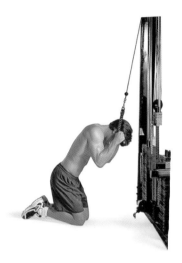

1. Kneel in front of a high-pulley cable and grab a rope attachment with both hands. Position your hands either by your ears (palms facing in) or just below your chin (palms touching the top of your chest).

2. Keeping your hands locked in place, slowly curl yourself down and forward. Start by drawing your chin towards your chest, then letting your shoulders and back follow. Curl down as far as you comfortably can, then slowly reverse the motion.

3. After each repetition done in this way, curl yourself down while twisting either to the left or to the right. Alternate sides on each repetition to work your obliques.

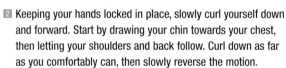

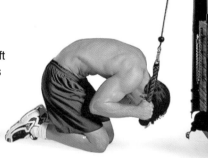

TORSO ROTATION

Stand with your right shoulder facing the machine. Reach your left arm across your face and grab the handle, then place your right hand on top of your left hand. Rotate your torso to your left as you draw your arms across and down. Once your hands are above your left thigh, slowly return to the starting position. Switch sides and repeat.

LOW PULLEY CRUNCH

■ **Targets:** Rectus Abdominis, Obliques

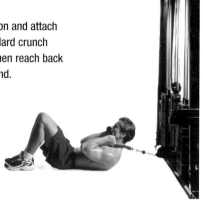

▣ Place a mat in front of a low-pulley station and attach a rope to the cable. Lie back in the standard crunch position, your head towards the pulley, then reach back and grab one end of the rope in each hand.

▣ Tuck your fists by your chest and curl.

TRAINER'S TIP

This variation is ideal for lighter men who need to add the right amount of resistance to thoroughly work their abs.

WEIGHTED CRUNCH

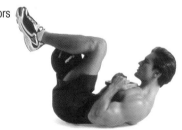

■ **Targets:** Rectus Abdominis, Obliques, Hip Flexors

▣ Lie flat on your back with your knees bent and your feet flat on the floor. Place a light medicine ball between your knees and squeeze it so it stays in place throughout the exercise.

▣ Hold a light weight plate (2.5 to 5 kilograms to start) in your hands. Slowly draw your knees up towards your chest while simultaneously curling your head and shoulders off the ground.

▣ Pause, then slowly lower your legs and upper body back to the floor, or just above the floor to keep constant tension on your rectus abdominis.

PARTNER UP

Instead of a weight plate, hold a medicine ball at your chest, keeping your elbows out to your sides. Get your workout partner to stand in front of you. As you curl up, throw the ball to your partner. Ask him to lightly toss the ball back at your chest so you can catch it, pull it back to your body and then curl back down.

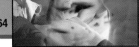

MEDICINE BALL CRUNCH

■ **Targets:** Rectus Abdominis, Obliques

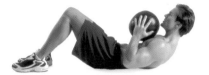

1. Lie with your feet flat on the floor, knees bent at a 90-degree angle.

2. Instead of placing your hands along-side your head, hold a medicine ball against your chest with both hands. This adds resistance more comfortably than holding a weight plate.

3. Slowly curl up, and then lower yourself back to the starting position.

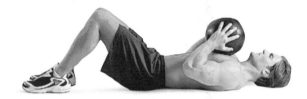

TWISTING LEGS-UP CRUNCH

■ **Targets:** Obliques, Rectus Abdominis

1. Lie on your back and raise your legs so that the soles of your feet point towards the ceiling.

2. Place your hands lightly behind your ears, elbows pointing out. Keeping your legs upright, slowly curl up and to the left.

3. Lower yourself and repeat to the right. Alternate from left to right throughout the set.

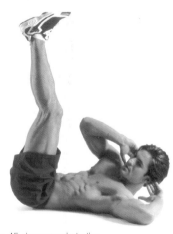

GET MORE

Start the move with your legs straight and suspended at a 45-degree angle to the floor. As you curl your upper body off the floor, simultaneously raise your legs until your feet point towards the ceiling. As you bring your head and shoulders back down to the floor, lower your legs back to a 45-degree angle.

PULSE TWIST

■ **Targets:** Obliques, Rectus Abdominis

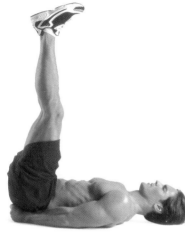

🔟 Lie on your back and tuck your hands under your pelvis, along the sides of your tailbone.

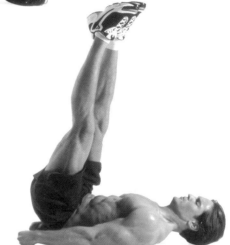

2️⃣ Keeping your legs straight and feet together, raise them so the soles of your feet point towards the ceiling and your buttocks lift a few centimetres off the floor. At the top of the move, twist your hips to the right so that your feet point to the left.

3️⃣ Lower your legs back to the starting position and repeat the move, this time twisting your hips to the left.

LEG ROTATION

Instead of twisting your hips at the top of the move, lower your buttocks to the floor, then slowly roll both legs to one side. Go as far as you comfortably can without losing your balance. Rotate your legs back up until they're above your hips and repeat the exercise, lowering your legs to the other side this time.

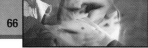

SIDE FLEX TWIST

■ **Targets:** Obliques, Rectus Abdominis

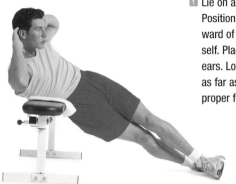

1 Lie on a weight bench on your right side. Position your left (top) leg slightly forward of your right leg to stabilize yourself. Place your hands behind your ears. Lower your shoulders and torso as far as you can while maintaining proper form.

2 Contracting your obliques, slowly raise your torso from the bench, twisting left. Repeat on the opposite side.

BARBELL ROLLOUT

■ **Targets:** All Mid-body Muscles

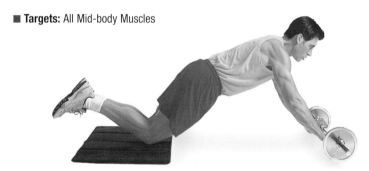

1 Start on your knees. Set a barbell slightly in front of your body. Grab the barbell with your hands about shoulder-width apart. Contract your abs, and then slowly roll the barbell forwards as far as you can without arching your back.

2 Slowly roll back to the starting position, keeping your abs contracted.

TRAINER'S TIP

Keep your body in the down position. Don't let your back sag or allow any part of your chest or upper body to touch the ground. Repeat.

REVERSE WOODCHOPPER

■ **Targets:** All Mid-body Muscles

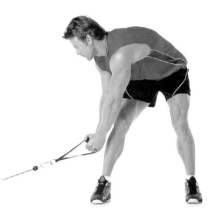

1 Attach a stirrup handle to a low-pulley cable, grab it with both hands, and stand with your right side facing the cable station and your feet shoulder-width apart. Bend over and hold the handle with both hands just outside your right calf muscle. Your shoulders will be rotated towards the cable machine. Straighten your arms and keep them straight throughout the whole movement.

2 Pull the handle up and across your torso as you straighten your body and twist your shoulders to the left. Your right arm will end up in front of your face, the handle at the same height as your ear.

3 Pause, then slowly return to the starting position. Finish the repetitions on this side, then switch sides to complete the set.

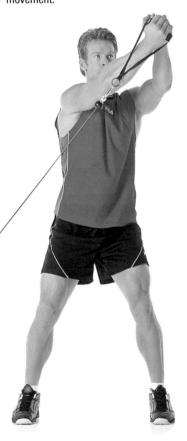

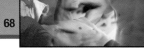

SAXON SIDE BEND

■ **Targets:** Obliques, Shoulders, Back

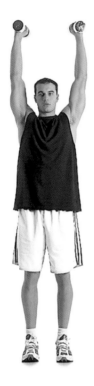

1 Grab a pair of lightweight dumbbells with an overhand grip and hold them overhead, in line with your shoulders, with your elbows slightly bent.

2 Keep your back straight and slowly bend directly to your left side as far as possible without twisting your upper body.

3 Pause, return to an upright position, then bend to your right side as far as possible.

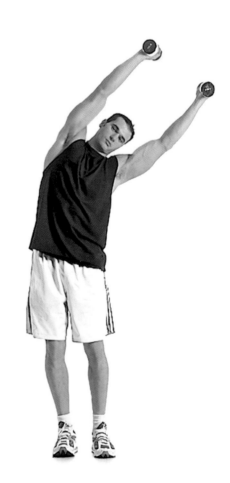

WORK WITH GRAVITY

This over-the-head dumbbell side bend forces your obliques — the muscles on the sides of your waist — to work extra hard. Because you're holding the weights over your head instead of at your sides, the lift works your shoulders and back as well. As a result, you exercise three muscle groups in one quick move.

No time for a total body workout? Do two or three sets of six to ten repetitions on each side.

THE BURNER

■ **Targets:** Obliques, Rectus Abdominis

1 Grab a dumbbell in your right hand with an overhand grip and hold it at arm's length in front of your right thigh.

2 Stand on your left leg, holding your right foot about 30 centimetres off the floor.

3 Reach down and touch the dumbbell to the floor on the outside of your left foot by leaning forwards and twisting your torso to the left.

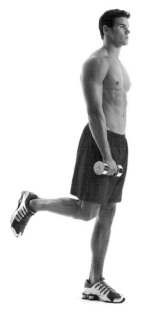

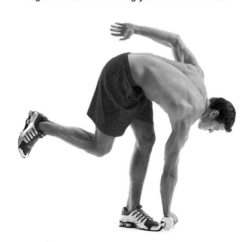

4 Stand up and reach behind your right shoulder with the dumbbell as you bend your left knee and twist to your right. Keep your right arm nearly straight, and your right foot a few centimetres off the floor.

5 Pause, then lean forwards and repeat.

TRAINER'S TIP

This move strengthens your abdominals at their weakest angle – a key to improving sports performance – while reducing your risk of knee injuries.

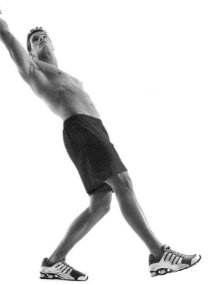

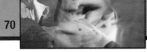

SITUP

■ **Targets:** Rectus Abdominis, Obliques, Hip Flexors

1 Lie on your back with knees bent and
feet flat on the floor. Hold a light
weight on your chest with both hands.

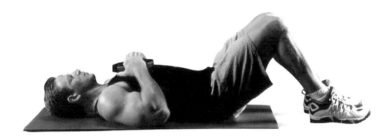

2 Inhale as you curl your torso off the
floor.

3 Return to the starting position and
perform the next rep without resting
your back on the floor.

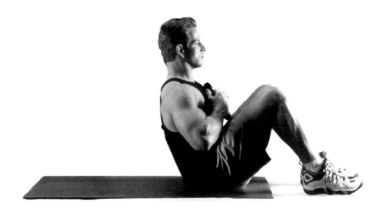

RUSSIAN TWIST

■ **Targets:** Obliques

1 Sit on the floor with your knees bent and your feet flat on the floor. Hold your arms straight out in front of your chest with your palms facing down. Lean back so your torso is at a 45-degree angle to the floor. Twist to the left as far as you can and pause.

2 Reverse the movement and twist all the way back to the right as far as you can. As you get stronger, hold a light weight in your hands as you do this.

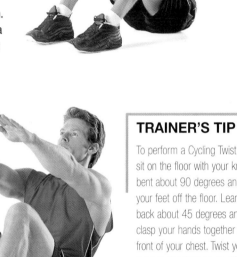

TRAINER'S TIP

To perform a Cycling Twist, sit on the floor with your knees bent about 90 degrees and your feet off the floor. Lean back about 45 degrees and clasp your hands together in front of your chest. Twist your torso to the right as you lift your left knee towards your chest. Then twist to your left as you lower your left knee and raise your knee in a cycling motion. That's one rep.

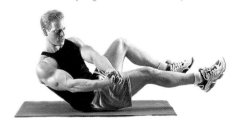

TOE TOUCH

■ **Targets:** Rectus Abdominis

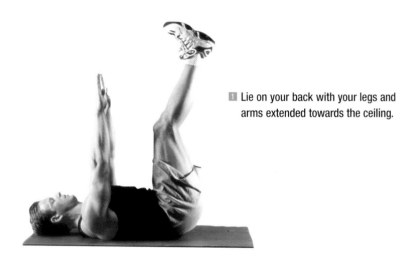

1 Lie on your back with your legs and arms extended towards the ceiling.

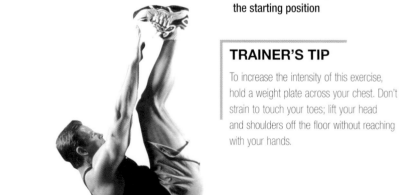

2 Slowly lift your head and shoulders. As you curl up, reach as high as you can with your fingers; then return to the starting position

TRAINER'S TIP

To increase the intensity of this exercise, hold a weight plate across your chest. Don't strain to touch your toes; lift your head and shoulders off the floor without reaching with your hands.

MODIFIED V-SIT

■ **Targets:** Rectus Abdominis, Hip Flexors, Obliques

1 Lie on your back with legs straight, heels a couple of centimetres off the floor, and hands at your sides.

2 Keeping your arms parallel to the floor, lift your torso and legs so they form a 'V' shape. As you come up, bend your knees and pull them up to your chest; then return to the starting position.

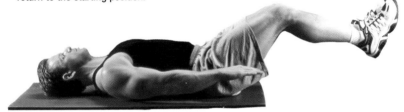

TRAINER'S TIP

To make this difficult move even more challenging keep your heels and upper back off the floor between repetitions, or try holding a light weight across your chest.

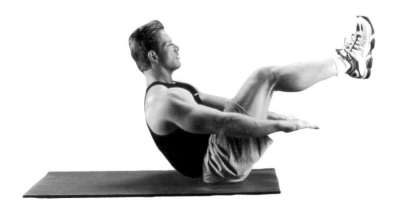

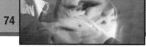

BRIDGE

■ **Targets:** All Mid-body Muscles

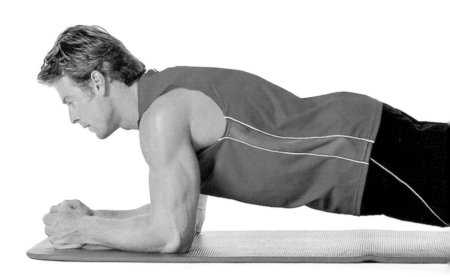

TWO-POINT BRIDGE

■ **Targets:** All Mid-body Muscles

1 Get into the standard press-up position.

2 Lift your right hand and your left leg off the floor at the same time (see right). Hold for 3 to 5 seconds. That's one repetition.

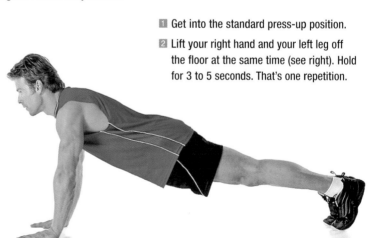

1. Start to get into a press-up position, but bend your elbows and rest your weight on your forearms instead of your hands. Your body should form a straight line from your shoulders to your ankles.

2. Pull in your abdominals; imagine you're trying to move your belly button back to your spine. Hold this for 20 to 30 seconds, breathing steadily.

3. Release, then repeat for another 20 to 30 seconds. That equals two complete sets. As you build endurance, you can do one 60-second set instead of two shorter ones.

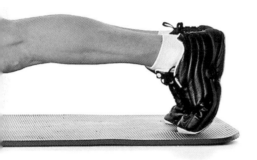

3. Return to the starting position, then repeat, lifting your left hand and your right leg this time. Alternate until you've completed all of your repetitions. Make sure you do an equal number with each hand and leg.

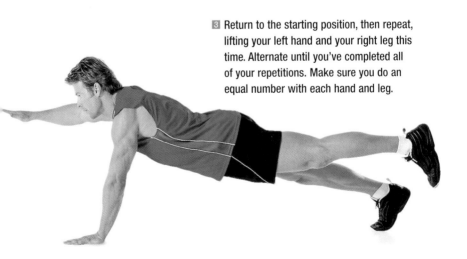

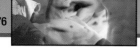

PRESS-UP BRIDGE

■ **Targets:** All Mid-body Muscles

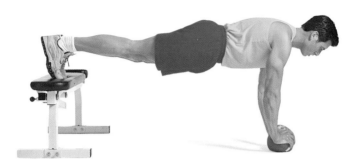

Position yourself in a press-up position on a weight bench so your hands are flat on the floor and your toes are on the bench. To increase the difficulty, you may place your hands on a football or medicine ball. Contract your abs and hold for 20 seconds. Continue to breathe without relaxing your abs. Rest, and then repeat. The goal is to work up to two 60-second sets.

SWISS BALL BRIDGE

■ **Targets:** All Mid-body Muscles

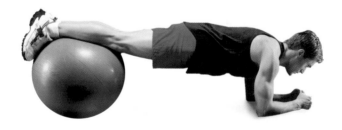

Position yourself on a Swiss ball so that your shins are on the top of the ball and you're supporting your weight on your forearms. Keep your neck straight – don't look up. Contract your abs and hold for 20 seconds. Continue to breathe without relaxing your abs. Rest, and then repeat. The goal is to work up to two 60-second sets.

SWISS BALL STABILITY POSE

■ **Targets:** All Mid-body Muscles

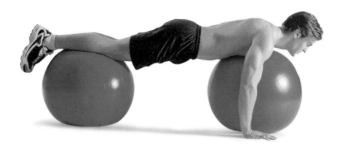

1 Lie face down across two Swiss balls. Your body should be straight, with just your chest lying on the first ball and your knees and shins resting on the other ball.

2 With your feet spaced about 30 to 45 centimetres apart, place your hands on the floor for balance and hold this position for 60 seconds.

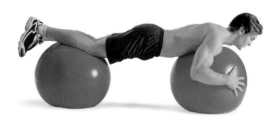

GET MORE

As the stability pose becomes easy, place your hands on the sides of the ball. For a greater challenge, try reaching your arms out to the sides or straightening them in front of your head. Moving your feet closer together so they touch also increases the difficulty.

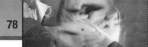

HANGING LEG RAISE

■ **Targets:** Rectus Abdominis, Hip Flexors, Obliques

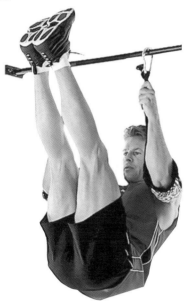

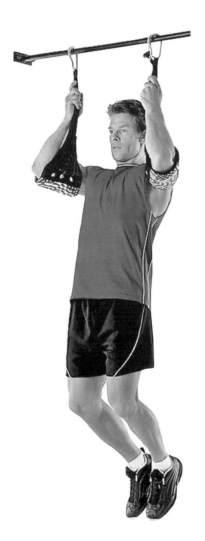

1 Grasp a chinup bar with an overhand grip and hang from it at arm's length, with your knees slightly bent. If you have elbow straps, hang from them.

2 Without bending your legs any more, lift your knees as close to your chest as possible by rounding your back and curling your hips towards your ribcage.

3 Pause, then slowly lower your legs to the starting position.

OBLIQUE HANGING LEG RAISE

■ **Targets:** Rectus Abdominis, Hip Flexors, Obliques

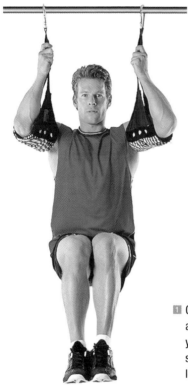

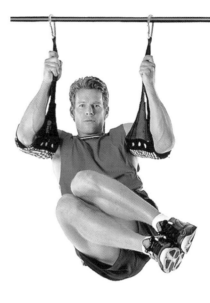

1 Grasp a chinup bar with an overhand grip and hang from it at arm's length, with your knees slightly bent. If you have elbow straps, hang from them. Then raise your legs until your knees are bent at 90 degrees.

2 Keep your knees bent and lift your left hip towards your left armpit, until your lower legs are nearly parallel to the floor.

3 Pause, then return to the starting position and lift your right hip towards your right armpit. That's one repetition.

TRAINER'S TIP

The Oblique Hanging Leg Raise is an advanced exercise that may cause lower-back pain, particularly if you have a pre-existing back condition. If you experience discomfort, do not perform this exercise. Instead, try the Seated Jackknife or Swiss Ball Press-up/Jackknife on pages 56–57. Both exercises target the lower abdominal muscles without straining the lower back.

Chest, Back and Arms

Build a powerful upper body to go with your lean, chiselled abs

BENCH PRESS

■ **Targets:** Pectoralis Major, Triceps

1 Lie on your back on a weight bench. Grab the bar with a wide, overhand grip. Slowly lower the bar to your chest.

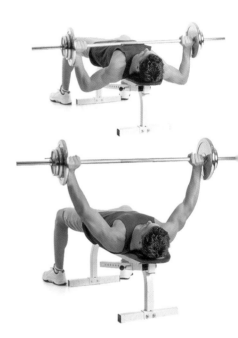

2 Slowly push the bar straight up until your arms are extended. The barbell should be positioned over your chin.

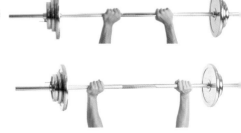

Close Grip
Positioning your hands directly above your shoulders involves your triceps and deltoids in the exercise.

Medium Grip
With hands positioned just beyond shoulder width, your chest becomes the primary target.

SHOULDER PRESS

■ **Targets:** Deltoids, Triceps, Lower Trapezius

1 Grab a pair of dumbbells and sit on a bench. Hold the dumbbells at the sides of your shoulders, with your arms bent and palms facing each other.

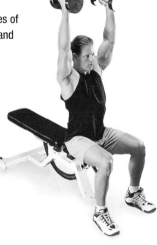

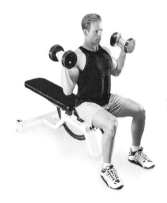

2 Push the weights straight overhead, pause, then slowly lower them.

BICEPS CURL

■ **Targets:** Biceps, Deltoids

1 Stand with your head up and your legs straight. Hold a pair of dumbbells with an underhand grip at arm's length in front of your body.

2 Curl the dumbbells up at the same time; your palms should be facing up when you are at the end of the movement.

TRAINER'S TIPS

• Do not swing your arms or elbows. Keep your arms close to your sides throughout the movement.

• For a more rigorous exercise, perform a barbell biceps curl with your back against the wall. Try to keep your shoulder blades pressed against the wall for the best results.

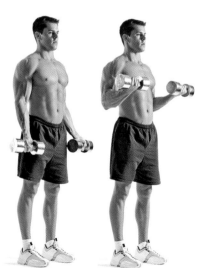

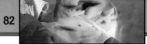

DIPS

■ **Targets:** Triceps, Pectoralis Major, Front Shoulders

1 Grab the parallel bars and lift yourself so your arms are fully extended.

2 Bend your elbows and slowly lower your body until your upper arms are parallel to the floor.

3 Pause, then push yourself back up to the starting position.

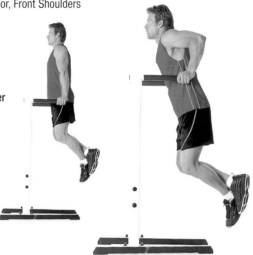

LYING TRICEPS EXTENSION

■ **Targets:** Triceps

1 Lie on your back on a weight bench. Hold a straight or EZ-curl bar with your arms extended and your hands 15 to 30 centimetres apart in an overhand grip.

2 Lower the barbell by bending your elbows until the bar is at the top of your forehead. Pause, and then return to the starting position.

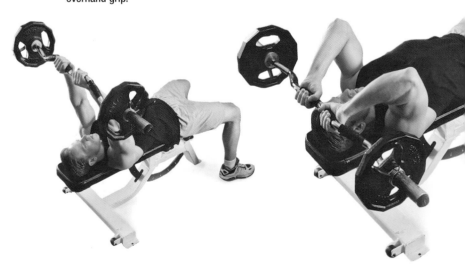

POWER CLEAN AND PRESS

■ **Targets:** Deltoids, Trapezius, Triceps

1 Grab a pair of dumbbells and stand with your feet shoulder-width apart. Hold the dumbbells straight down at arm's length, palms facing your thighs.

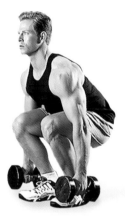

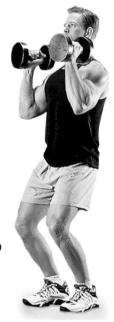

2 In one motion, pull the dumbbells up to your shoulders as you dip your body down to 'catch' them.

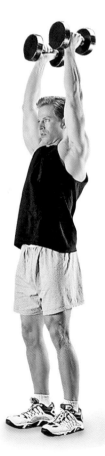

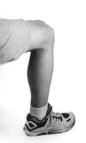

3 Push up to a standing position, then press the weights overhead.

4 Pause, then lower the weights to shoulder level and return to the starting position.

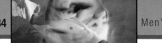

BARBELL BENT-OVER ROW

■ **Targets:** Latissimus Dorsi, Trapezius, Rear Deltoids, Biceps

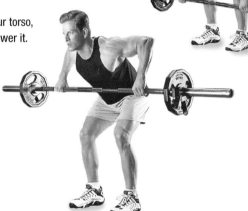

1 Grab a barbell with an overhand grip that's just beyond shoulder width, and hold it down at arm's length. Stand with your feet shoulder-width apart and knees slightly bent. Bend at the hips, lowering your torso about 45 degrees, and let the bar hang straight down from your shoulders.

2 Pull the bar up to your torso, pause, then slowly lower it.

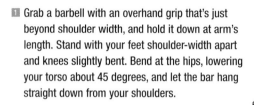

DUMBBELL UPRIGHT ROW

■ **Targets:** Deltoids, Trapezius

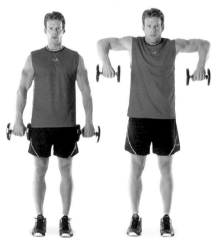

1 Grab a pair of dumbbells with an overhand grip and stand with your feet shoulder-width apart, your knees slightly bent. Let the dumbbells hang at arm's length next to the outside of your thighs, thumbs pointed towards each other.

2 Bending your elbows, lift your upper arms straight out to the sides and pull the dumbbells straight up, until your upper arms are parallel to the floor and the dumbbells are just below chest level. (You'll look like a scarecrow.)

3 Pause, then return to the starting position.

CABLE ROW

■ **Targets:** Latissimus Dorsi, Trapezius, Rear Deltoids, Biceps

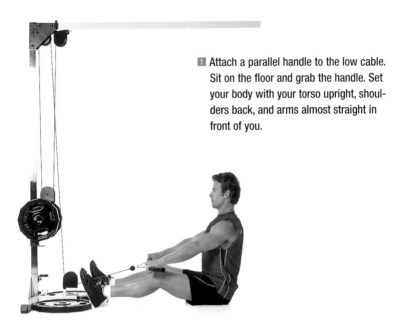

1 Attach a parallel handle to the low cable. Sit on the floor and grab the handle. Set your body with your torso upright, shoulders back, and arms almost straight in front of you.

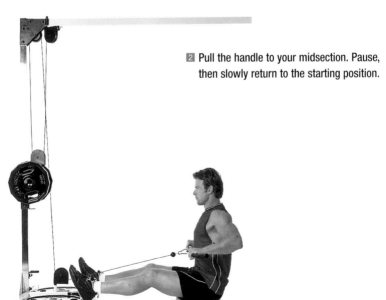

2 Pull the handle to your midsection. Pause, then slowly return to the starting position.

LAT PULL-DOWN

■ **Targets:** Latissimus Dorsi, Trapezius, Biceps

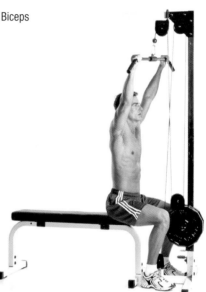

1. Grab the bar overhead with an overhand grip (palms facing away from you), hands just beyond shoulder width.

2. Sit on the seat and, keeping your head and back straight, slowly pull the bar to the top of your chest. Pause, then let the bar rise back above your head – resisting the weight as you go – until your arms are straight again, but be sure to keep your elbows unlocked.

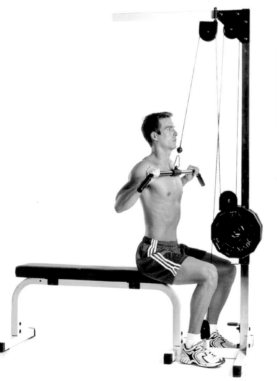

REVERSE YOUR GRIP

Try grabbing the straight bar at the lat pull-down station with an underhand grip. This variation still builds your upper-back muscles while letting the biceps help curl the bar at the bottom of the move. Also, this position forces the forearms, wrists and hands to work harder than they have to in most back exercises, helping you develop a stronger grip at the same time.

Legs

Complete your physique with a strong, muscular lower body

DUMBBELL STEPUP

■ **Targets:** Quadriceps, Gluteals, Hamstrings

1 Grab a pair of dumbbells and stand in front of a bench or step that's 30 to 45 centimetres high.

2 Step up onto the bench with your right foot and push off with your right heel to lift the rest of your body onto the step. Step down with your left foot first, then your right.

3 Finish the set with your right leg, then repeat the set with your left leg, stepping up with your left and back with your right.

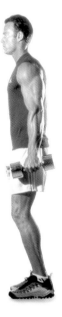

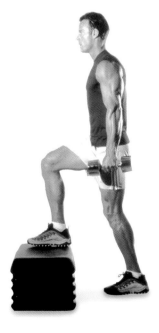

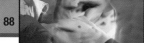

JUMP SHRUG

■ **Targets:** Upper Trapezius, Gripping Muscles, Calves

1 Grab a pair of dumbbells and hold them at your sides, arms extended, palms towards your thighs. Set your feet shoulder-width apart, and bend your knees slightly.

2 Bend your knees a bit further, then jump as high as you can, simultaneously shrugging your shoulders and pulling your toes upwards, towards your shins.

3 Land with your knees bent to absorb the impact. Pause, reset your body and repeat.

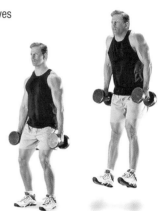

TRAINER'S TIP

On the jump squat and jump shrug, light weights go a long way. Start with a quarter to a third of the weight you'd use without a jump.

JUMP SQUAT

■ **Targets:** Quadriceps, Hamstrings, Calves, Gluteals, Lower Back

1 Hold a barbell across the back of your shoulders and stand with your feet shoulder-width apart. Sit back into a squat.

2 Jump up to the starting position.

3 Land with your knees bent to absorb the impact. Pause, reset your body and repeat.

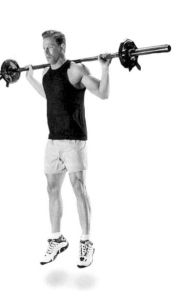

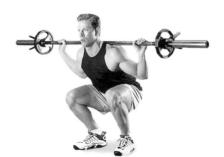

BARBELL SQUAT

■ **Targets:** Entire Lower Body

[1] Place a barbell across your shoulders and step back from the squat rack. Set your feet shoulder-width apart and place your hands just beyond shoulder-width apart on the bar.

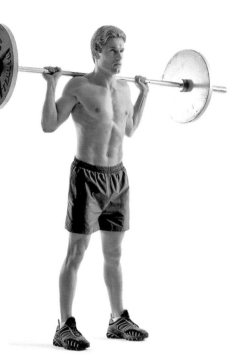

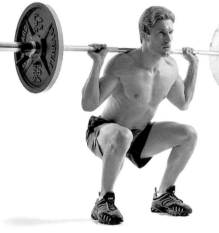

[2] Bend at the knees and hips, as if you were sitting down in a chair, and lower your body until your thighs are parallel to the floor.

[3] Pause, then return to the starting position.

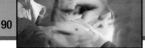

WALKING LUNGE

■ **Targets:** Quadriceps, Hamstrings, Gluteals

1 Grab a pair of dumbbells and hold them at your sides. Stand with your feet hip-width apart at one end of your exercise room or living room.

2 Lunge forwards with your right leg, bending the knee 90 degrees. Your left knee should also bend and almost touch the floor.

3 Stand and bring your left foot up next to your right, then repeat with the left leg lunging forward. That's one repetition. Continue until you've completed half your repetitions in this direction. Turn and do the same number of walking lunges back to your starting point.

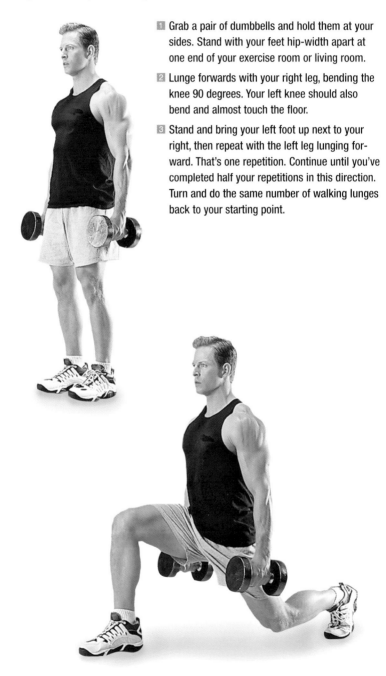

WINDMILL LUNGE

■ **Targets:** Quadriceps, Hamstrings, Gluteals

1 Stand holding a pair of dumbbells at your sides, feet hip-width apart. Lunge forwards with your right leg until your left knee is bent 90 degrees. Step back to the starting position.

2 Now lunge out at a 45-degree angle with your right leg, then return. Lunge sideways with your right leg, then return. Lunge backwards at a 45-degree angle with your right leg, then return. Lunge straight back with your right leg, then return.

3 Now step straight back with your left leg, then return. Lunge back at a 45-degree angle with your left leg, then return. Lunge sideways with your left leg, then return. Lunge forwards at a 45-degree angle with your left leg, then return. Lunge forwards with your left leg, then return. That's one complete set.

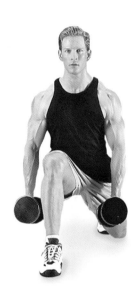

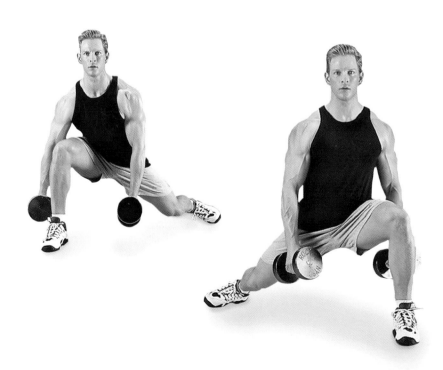

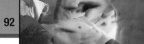

LYING LEG CURL

■ **Targets:** Hamstrings

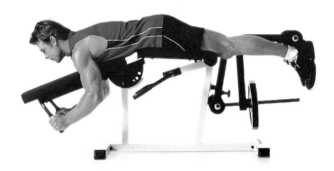

1 Lie face down on a leg-curl machine with the pads against your lower legs, above your heel and below your calf muscles.

2 Without raising your body off the pads, bend your legs at the knees and pull the weight towards you as far as you can.

3 Pause, then slowly return to the starting position.

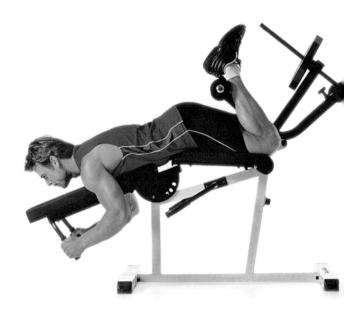

CALF RAISE

■ **Targets:** Gastrocnemius, Soleus

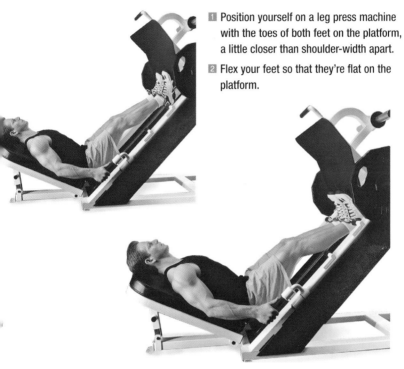

1 Position yourself on a leg press machine with the toes of both feet on the platform, a little closer than shoulder-width apart.

2 Flex your feet so that they're flat on the platform.

LEG EXTENSION

■ **Targets:** Quadriceps

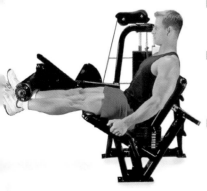

1 Sit on the leg extension machine, making sure that the backs of your knees are supported by the seat.

2 Holding the machine handles, slowly extend your legs straight out in front of you, pause and then slowly return to the starting position

3 Move the lever forwards by extending your knees until your legs are straight. Return the lever to the original position by bending your knees. Repeat.

BACK EXTENSION

■ **Targets:** Hamstrings, Gluteals, Lower Back

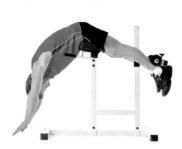

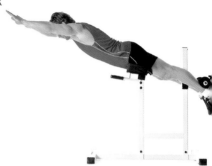

1 Position yourself in a back-extension station and hook your feet under the leg anchor. Hold your arms straight out in front of you. Your body should form a straight line from your hands to your hips. Lower your torso, allowing your lower back to round, until it's just short of perpendicular to the floor.

2 Raise your upper body until it's slightly above parallel to the floor. At this point, you should have a slight arch in your back, and your shoulder blades should be pulled together at the back.

3 Pause for a second or two, then repeat.

TWISTING BACK EXTENSION

■ **Targets:** Hamstrings, Gluteals, Lower Back, Obliques

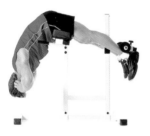

1 Position yourself in a back-extension station and hook your feet under the leg anchor. Place your fingers behind your ears.

2 Lower your upper body, allowing your lower back to round, until it's just short of perpendicular to the floor.

3 Raise and twist your upper body until it's slightly above parallel to the floor and facing left.

4 Pause, then lower your torso and repeat, this time twisting to the right. That's one repetition.

INDEX

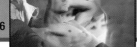